I0482611

TATTOO
*The Invaluable Compendium
for Dermatologists*

TATTOO
The Invaluable Compendium for Dermatologists

Editors

Shashikumar BM MD (DVL) FIADVL (Dermatopathology)
Associate Professor
Department of Dermatology,
Venereology and Leprosy
Mandya Institute of Medical Sciences
Mandya, Karnataka, India

Savitha AS MD DNB FRGUHS (Dermatosurgery)
Assistant Professor
Department of Dermatology,
Venereology and Leprosy
Sapthagiri Institute of Medical Sciences and Research Centre
Bengaluru, Karnataka, India

R Raghunatha Reddy MD DNB FRGUHS (Dermatosurgery)
Professor
Consultant Dermatologist and Dermatosurgeon
Dr Raghu's Mathapitha Skin Clinic
Bengaluru, Karnataka, India

Foreword

Nicolas Kluger MD PhD

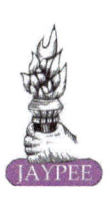

JAYPEE

The Health Sciences Publisher
New Delhi | London | Panama

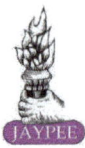 **Jaypee Brothers Medical Publishers (P) Ltd**

Headquarters
Jaypee Brothers Medical Publishers (P) Ltd.
4838/24, Ansari Road, Daryaganj
New Delhi 110 002, India
Phone: +91-11-43574357
Fax: +91-11-43574314
E-mail: jaypee@jaypeebrothers.com

Overseas Offices
J.P. Medical Ltd.
83, Victoria Street, London
SW1H 0HW (UK)
Phone: +44-20 3170 8910
Fax: +44(0)20 3008 6180
E-mail: info@jpmedpub.com

Jaypee-Highlights Medical Publishers Inc.
City of Knowledge, Bld. 235, 2nd Floor, Clayton
Panama City, Panama
Phone: +1 507-301-0496
Fax: +1 507-301-0499
E-mail: cservice@jphmedical.com

Jaypee Brothers Medical Publishers (P) Ltd.
17/1-B, Babar Road, Block-B, Shaymali
Mohammadpur, Dhaka-1207
Bangladesh
Mobile: +08801912003485
E-mail: jaypeedhaka@gmail.com

Jaypee Brothers Medical Publishers (P) Ltd.
Bhotahity, Kathmandu, Nepal
Phone: +977-9741283608
E-mail: kathmandu@jaypeebrothers.com

Website: www.jaypeebrothers.com
Website: www.jaypeedigital.com

TATTOO: The Invaluable Compendium for Dermatologists

First Edition: **2017**
ISBN: 978-93-5270-078-3
Printed at

Dedicated to

All our patients from whom we have learnt

CONTRIBUTORS

Savitha AS
MD DNB FRGUHS (Dermatosurgery)
Assistant Professor
Department of Dermatology,
Venereology and Leprosy
Sapthagiri Institute of Medical
Sciences and Research Centre
Bengaluru, Karnataka, India

Sanjeev J Aurangabadkar MD
Consultant Dermatologist
Skin and Laser Clinic
Hyderabad, Andhra Pradesh, India

Shashikumar BM
MD (DVL) FIADVL (Dermatopathology)
Associate Professor
Department of Dermatology
Venereology and Leprosy
Mandya Institute of Medical Sciences
Mandya, Karnataka, India

Lakshmi DV DVD FRGUHS
Consultant Dermatologist
Bengaluru, Karnataka, India

Shilpa K MD FRGUHS (Dermatosurgery)
Assistant Professor
Department of Dermatology,
Venereology and Leprosy
Bangalore Medical College and
Research Institute
Bengaluru, Karnataka, India

Kavya M MD
Assistant Professor
Department of Dermatology,
Venereology and Leprosy
Mandya Institute of Medical Sciences
Mandya, Karnataka, India

Sukesh MS MD DNB FIADVL FISD
Consultant Dermatologist and
Trichologist
Bengaluru, Karnataka, India.

Umashankar Nagaraju MD (DVL)
Professor
Department of Dermatology,
Venereology and Leprosy
Rajarajeswari Medical College
and Hospital
Bengaluru, Karnataka, India

Smitha Prabhu S MD (DVL)
Associate Professor
Department of Dermatology,
Venereology and Leprosy
Kasturba Medical College
Manipal University
Manipal, Karnataka, India

R Raghunatha Reddy
MD DNB FRGUHS (Dermatosurgery)
Professor
Consultant Dermatologist and
Dermatosurgeon
Dr Raghu's Mathapitha Skin Clinic
Bengaluru, Karnataka, India

Sujit Shanshanwal
Resident
Department of Dermatology,
Venereology and Leprosy
Lokmanya Tilak Municipal Medical
College and Sion Hospital
Mumbai, Maharashtra, India

FOREWORD

When Professor Shashikumar from the Mandya Institute of Medical Sciences, Mandya, Karnataka, India contacted me to write this foreword for this book titled *Tattoo—The Invaluable Compendium for Dermatologists*, I must admit that my knowledge and vision of tattooing in India were the ones of a French Epinal imprint, traditionalist and naïve—a roadside tattoo artist in the 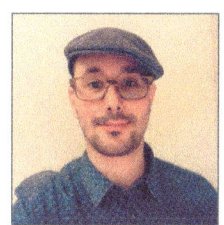 middle of a village in rural and remote areas of India, tattooing dozens of young girls and women, who would develop years later inoculation leprosy or tuberculosis on their tattoos.

But no, modern tattooing is global, irrespective of age, gender, social classes, religion or continents. Nowadays, Indian physicians have to face the same issues regarding tattooing as we do in Western countries—tattoo infection, ink allergies, amateur backyard tattooists or tattoo removal requests.

For this first-ever book on tattoos in India, Professor Shashikumar did a real tour de force. From epidemiology to tattoo-removal techniques, the book covers all the fields of permanent and temporary tattooing in India with updated data and it is abundantly illustrated with original clinical and histopathological photographs from Indian collections.

Needless to say that this book will be of an invaluable help not only for any Indian dermatologist or resident in dermatology, but also for general practitioners, infectious specialists dealing with issues related to tattooing. It may be of interest for Indian tattooists to improve their work. For Western physicians, this book is an invitation to discover the specificities and faces of Indian tattooing.

Paris, April 22nd, 2017

Nicolas Kluger MD PhD
Department of Dermatology, Venereology and Allergology
Helsinki University Central Hospital and University of Helsinki
Helsinki, Finland
Tattoo Complications Consultation
Department of Dermatology
Bichat-Claude Bernard Hospital
Assistance Publique des Hôpitaux de Paris
Paris, France
Vice-President
European Society of Tattoo and Pigment Research (ESTP)
Denmark

PREFACE

Think Before You Ink!

Tattooing is a very old practice, which involves insertion of ink pigment of the desired color into the dermis. It is practiced worldwide, across all cultures and is becoming increasingly common in India. Furthermore, it is becoming more prevalent among rural youngsters of India due to increased enthusiasm towards newer fashion trends exposing to increased risks and complications associated with it. There is a paucity of literature on tattoo except for a few case reports and case series.

Since there is no book published from India on tattoos, so we are presenting for our readers the first-ever book on this topic. It covers history of tattoo, types of tattooing, psychosocial aspects and uses of tattooing in details. The authors have tried to cover tattoo complications and its management, and various modalities for the removal of tattoo, including lasers in details. Few chapters on safe tattoo alternative and regulations on tattoo have been covered extensively.

Most of the complications associated with tattooing or tattoo removal have been described with relevant photographs. Also, various tips and tricks of laser tattoo removal have been described in a simple and comprehensive way.

We hope this book will be a valuable reference for the researchers, health professionals, and policy experts, and a useful resource for all those who have interest in tattoos.

Shashikumar BM
Savitha AS
R Raghunatha Reddy

ACKNOWLEDGMENTS

We are grateful to all the authors who have contributed sincerely. We would like to express our gratitude to Dr Nicolas Kluger from whom we got inspiration. We thank him for his kind foreword.

We sincerely appreciate Dr Harish MR, Professor and Head, Department of Dermatology, Mandya Institute of Medical Sciences (MIMS), Mandya, Karnataka, India, who encouraged us to take up this project.

We would like to thank all the staff and postgraduates of the Department of Dermatology, MIMS, Mandya for helping us in editing the proof.

We would also like to thank Mr Jitendar P Vij (Group Chairman), Mr Ankit Vij (Group President), Ms Chetna Malhotra Vohra (Associate Director-Content Strategy), Ms Kritika Dua (Development Editor), and the entire team of Jaypee Brothers Medical Publishers, New Delhi, India for their outstanding efforts in bringing out this book in record time.

CONTENTS

Chapter 1

History and Epidemiology of Tattoo

Savitha AS, Lakshmi DV

INTRODUCTION

Skin was the first canvas for art. Tattooing is an ancient technique and human tattoos have been identified from ancient times, dating back even to the Stone Age 5,300 years.[1] Historical and archeological evidence show that tattooing was practiced throughout the world as indigenous cultures from every continent. The body marks by tattooing process acted to negotiate relationships between individuals and their society, nature, and the spiritual realm. Through their traditions, they have functioned to signal entry into adulthood, reflect social status, document martial achievement, demonstrate lineage and group affiliation, and to channel and direct preternatural forces.[2] In ancient cultures, the house served not only as a physical shelter but also as a border between the family and the outside world. People used items and rituals with magical or spiritual meanings to protect the front door which was seen as the most "fragile" opening of the house. Similar to this belief, the skin was often regarded as the border between the human body and the exterior world and the human body was also protected in fragile places with the help of permanent skin markings.[3] Hence, art of tattoo was not mere esthetic on body but beyond; an amalgamation of their life, culture, nature and afterlife.

ORIGIN OF THE TERMINOLOGY "TATTOO"

It is likely that the word "tattoo" is an onomatopoeia; that is, a word that sounds like the special sounds this technique makes. The word tattoo is English in origin and attributed to Captain Thomas Cook who wrote about his travels in Polynesia in 1766–1779. In a narrative referred to in the ship's log for *HMS Endeavour* on 29th July 1769, published in 1773 with the title

"Captain Cook's First Voyage", he explained the origin of the word as being an adaptation of the Polynesian word "tatow": *'Both sexes paint their bodies "tatow" as it is called in their language. This is done by inlaying the color of black under their skins in such a manner as to be indelible.'*[4] The term "tattooing" is derived from "tattau", a Tahitian word which translates essentially as "to mark" and is a process of implantation of permanent pigment granules in the skin.[5] Thus, the origin and historical meaning of the word "tattoo" is believed to have two derivations as follow: (i) "ta"—*striking something* (Samoan/Polynesian) (ii) "tatau"—*to mark something* (Tahitian).

The Latin word "Picti" was first used in a panegyric written by Eumenius in AD 297 which means "painted or tattooed" people. Roman military commanders used to describe the inhabitants of present day Scotland as the Picts, group of late Iron age and early medieval Celtic people, who terrified the Roman legions with their naked painted bodies from black or dark blue dye of woad leaves (cabbage plant of European origin) and drew complex war designs. Similarly, word Britons means "people of the designs".[6]

TATTOOING AS A CULTURE

Tattoos are known from ancient Egypt, from South America, as mentioned from Eskimos in Greenland and Canada, from Africa and the Pacific Ocean region, where they were very common. One of the major intentions of tattooing was to mark an individual as a part of a tribe known as *Tribal tattoos* (ethnic tattoos/clan markings or magic tattoos). In many cultures, tribal tattoos have been for men, women and children. Tattoos have often been carried out when a person reached a certain age, as a mark that the person has had a kind of confirmation of being included in the tribe's communal life and responsibility, or as a sign that the tattooed person was now to be considered as adult and sexually mature.[1]

Among the Maoris and Inuits, aborigines of New Zealand linear face tattoos were carried out by pricking pigment into the skin or inserting it with blackened threads and were known as *Moko style tattoos* (moko meaning to strike or tap). It was used as a form of identification with regards to rank, genealogy, tribal history, eligibility to marry, beauty and virility. Maori women were traditionally only allowed to be tattooed on their lips, around the chin, and sometimes the nostrils. While in Africa, they have most often been designed as linear body tattoos cut into the skin with the possible intention of scarification; in Asia there have been many different forms carried out using a variety of techniques and have been placed on very different parts of the body.[7] Hawaiians also celebrate specific tattoo Gods where in priests conducted tattooing.

Totem animal tattoos were also another common motif in primitive tattoos and animal is thought to have a special spiritual relationship with the bearer of tattoo and acts as a spirit guide.

Totem animals such as snakes, frogs, butterflies wolves or bears signified that the individual has taken on the physical prowess of that animal. In China, tattooing one's animal astrological symbol, such as the pig or the horse is thought to bring good fortune and images of Koi, carp or goldfish were thought to bring prosperity and wealth to the bearer.

TATTOO AND RELIGION

At about 1900 tattoos were disliked, disapproved of and not very prevalent in cultural circles in Europe as well as in the general population. In the old testament of the Bible, the book of Leviticus, verse 19:28 says: *"Ye shall not make any cuttings in your flesh for the dead, nor print any marks upon you: I am the LORD. I am the LORD".* The church and its missionaries around the world had argued against tattoos for centuries. At the Catholic council of Calcuth in Northumberland in 787, the church banned markings/tattoos on the skin. Also the Koran was and is against tattoos—the dead must not be marked. Tattoos were and are regarded as barbarian by the great religions. The Vikings, however, continued to believe in the Nordic gods and sometimes had tattoos.[7] The Roman Empire was also against tattoos and they were forbidden by Emperor Constantine (307–337). Therefore, hardly anyone in civilized Europe had tattoos until modern times, with the exception of certain purposes, such as marking criminals and foundlings.[8]

Tattoo as Symbol of Punishment

Branding tattoo describes a forced marking of individuals by a ruling authority. In the late middle ages, the practice focused on a differentiation between burning, pinching with a cold iron, and perforating the skin with needle stitches which were rubbed over with coal dust.[8] The purpose of these branding tattoos was usually to recognize what criminal act a person had committed, and besides being a physical punishment, this branding "marked" a criminal and led to his isolation within society.

Japanese tattoo artists developed the uniquely-Japanese traditional art tattoo art form, called *horimono*. Punitive tattoos were called *irezumi; ire*, or *ireru* means "to insert" (meaning the insertion of the pigment) and *zumi* means the ink itself. During the Edo period, tattooing as punishment, along with amputation of noses and ears, occurred between the eras of Kanbun (1661–1673) and Tenna (1681–1684). By 1720 punitive tattoos had replaced the amputation as part of the Kyōhō Reforms (1716–1736). These reforms, among other things, disassociated the tattooing from death penalty, instead imposing it as punishment for minor offenses.[9]

Modern Tattoo[10]

In the 1960s tattooing for art's sake alone became popular. Some people collect tattoos the way others collect antiques or works of art. In the 1970s, artists trained in traditional fine art disciplines began to embrace tattooing and brought innovative imagery and drawing techniques to the industry. Advances in electric needle guns and pigments provided them with new ranges of color, delicacy of detail and artistic possibilities. The cultural status of tattooing has steadily evolved from that of an anti-social activity in the 1940s to that of a trendy fashion statement in the year 2000. First adopted and flaunted by influential rock stars like the Rolling Stones in the early 1970s, tattooing had, by the late 1980s, become accepted by mainstream society. Cosmetic tattooing originated during '20s and '30s. Many artists started offering specialties such as moles and beauty marks rosy cheeks, permanent eyeliner and red lips to both male and female customers.

During the last 15 years, two distinct classes of tattoo business have emerged. The first is the "tattoo parlor" that glories in a sense of urban outlaw culture, advertises itself with garish exterior signage and offers less than sanitary surroundings. The second is the "tattoo art studio" that most frequently features custom and fine art designs, all of the features of a high-end beauty and "by-appointment" services only. Today's fine art tattoo studio draws the same kind of clients as a jewelry store, fashion boutique, or high-end antique shop.

HISTORY OF INDIAN TATTOOING[11]

In India, the practice of tattooing is a part of folk and tribal art. In the northern and northwestern regions, the tradition of tattooing has been prevalent among the Bhils and Santhals in central India, the Kanbis and Warlis in the Gujarat region, and among the Banjaras of Rajasthan. The young and old generations of Kanbi and Warli women practice tattooing on the forehead and cheeks. The characteristic symbol that is tattooed is of a tree and its leaves on the forehead. Tattoos are used both as a mark of beautification as well as a totem. Many women bear tattoo marks of the peepal tree or acasia tree, which is of religious significance in Hinduism. Men of these communities get tattooed the figure of the Hindu gods Hanuman, Krishna, the motif of "Om", etc. and their own names. The Rabaris, a wandering tribe of the Kutch, use tattooing as a practice of beautification of women. The women of this community wear small motifs on the throat, chin, and entire arms and on their hands (Fig. 1.1).

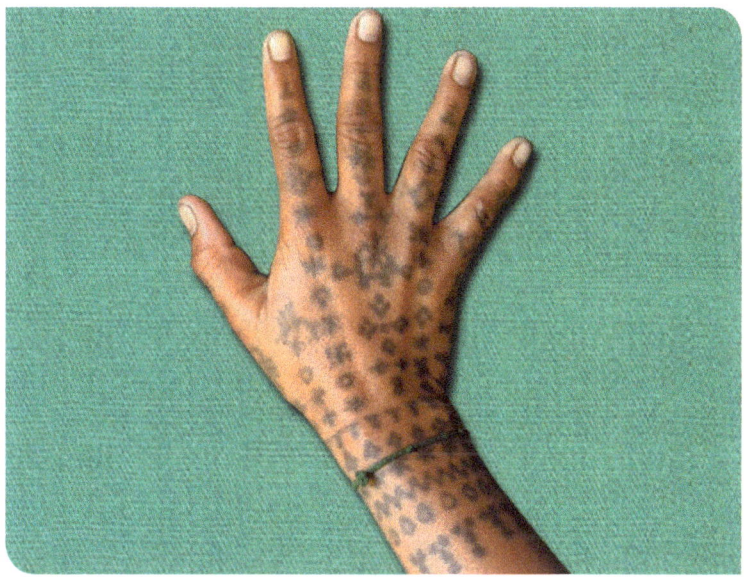

Fig. 1.1: Decorative tattoo on hands on Rabaris woman.
Source: Photo courtesy Meena Khadri. [online] Available at http://www.thebetterindia.com/58170/india-tattoo-tradition-history/

Amongst the Santhals of Bengal and Jharkhand, among women tattooing marks an important rite of passage for girls between the ages of 10 years and 11 years before their marriage. It is believed the painful experience prepares a girl for motherhood and gives her the strength to face the challenges of life. The men inscribe tattoos called "sikkas" on their forearms and wrists, named thus because they are usually the size of coins called "sikka". On the contrary, among Arunachal Pradesh's Apatani tribe tattooing its womenfolk was done to make them unattractive to rival tribes in neighboring districts, who might otherwise abduct their prettiest women. The Apatani tattooing procedure involved using thorns to cut the skin and soot mixed in animal fat to fill in the deep blue color. The wounds were then allowed to get infected so that the tattoos became larger, darker and clearer (Figs. 1.2 and 1.3).

The four prominent tribes namely the Gonds, Pardhans, Kolam, Korku and the nomadic Banjara tribe are the communities in Maharashtra that have been practicing tattooing. Moving southwards, the Malagasy-Nias-Dravidians of the Malabar Coast have been documented to be using "medicinal tattoos" as cures for physical ailments. The affected area of the body is believed to be cured by inscribing of a tattoo over it. Medicinal tattoos have been documented to be used in other communities in the world for treatment of joint-related conditions such as rheumatism.

In Nagas tribes, tattooing is linked to the identity and honor of the community. Most of the Naga tribes have been reported to have their faces

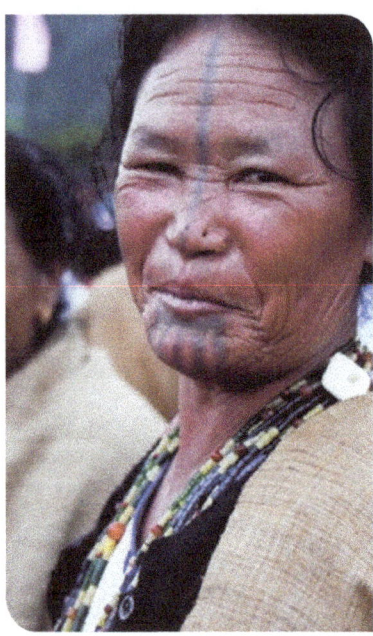

Fig. 1.2: Tattoo in Apatani woman.
Source: Photo courtesy Priyanka Verma. [online] Available at http://www.thebetterindia.com/58170/india-tattoo-tradition-history/.

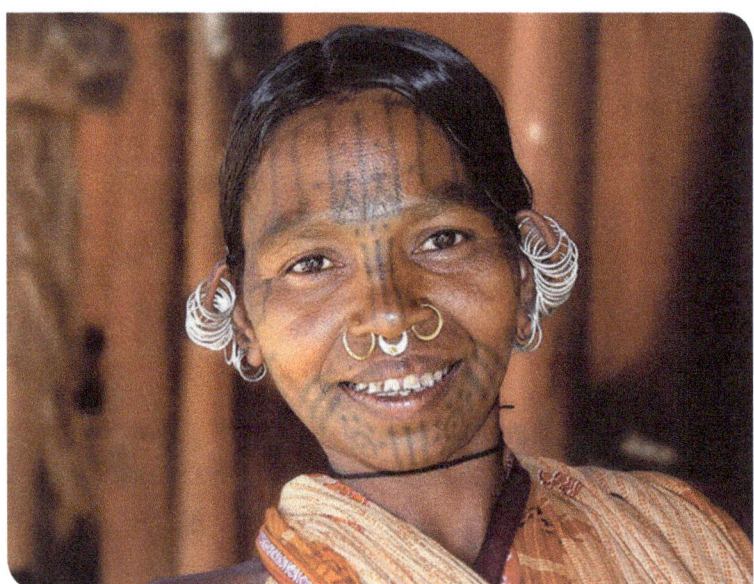

Fig. 1.3: Women of the Kutia Kondh tribe of Orissa, called the "the people of the spirit world", ink themselves with beautiful geometric facial tattoos; it is said these identifying marks ensure they recognize each other once they enter the spirit world.
Source: Photo courtesy Wikimedia Commons.

tattooed with distinctive marks with which one can identify what region of the hills they belong. Among Konyaks of Nagaland facial tattoo were used to commemorate their head-hunting expeditions. Facial tattooing was prevalent among the Noctes and Wanchos of Arunachal as well.

The tattooing of body parts for sexual expression also has a long history to realize significance of body adornment for sexual provocation. In central India, the Baiga female tattooed symbol of a peacock at the breast when a girl reaches puberty. It is strictly not tattooed until she is adolescent. Apart from this symbol, they also tattooed a symbol of basket (dauri) at their breast when a girl reaches puberty.[12] In Southern India, permanent tattoos are called *"pachakutharathu"*. They were very common, especially in Tamil Nadu, before 1980. The nomadic Korathi tattoo artists traveled the countryside in search of clients. The kollam, a sinuous labyrinthine design believed to ensnare evil beings, is inked on bodies to permanently keep them safe and secure until reunited with deceased ancestors in the afterlife.

Henna Tattoos

Henna tattoos are also used for centuries by Muslims and Hindus for cosmetic purposes. Henna has been used as a dye for the skin, hair and nails for over 4,000 years, and as an expression of body art, especially in Islamic and Hindu cultures in the Arab, African and Indian world. At events such as wedding parties, public celebrations, and religious ceremonies, henna is applied to the skin of the hands and feet. A range of products such as lemon, vinegar or tea leaves are used to prevent the deterioration of tattoos. It is a temporary tattoo that stains the skin in reddish-brown and disappears after 2 or 3 weeks by the natural process of renewal of the epidermis. These mehndi tattoos are used as a reminder of happiness and as a form of blessing for the wearer. In recent years, a new mode of henna application, the so-called temporary black henna tattoo, has become fashionable, especially among children, adolescents and young adults in western countries.[13,14] Black henna is the combination of henna proper and p-phenylenediamine (PPD).

TECHNIQUE OF TATTOOING

The classic tattoo pigment was simply whatever was at hand, which was typically soot; that is, carbon from burnt wood that was used as black pigment. Black was the dominant tattoo color, but sometimes pulverized colored minerals from nature were used for tattoos.[15] It is essential for classic tattoos to be permanent. By using a suitable technique or operation, the natural pigment was placed between the collagen fibers in the skin's corium (synonymous to dermis), which is a relatively stationary and mechanically

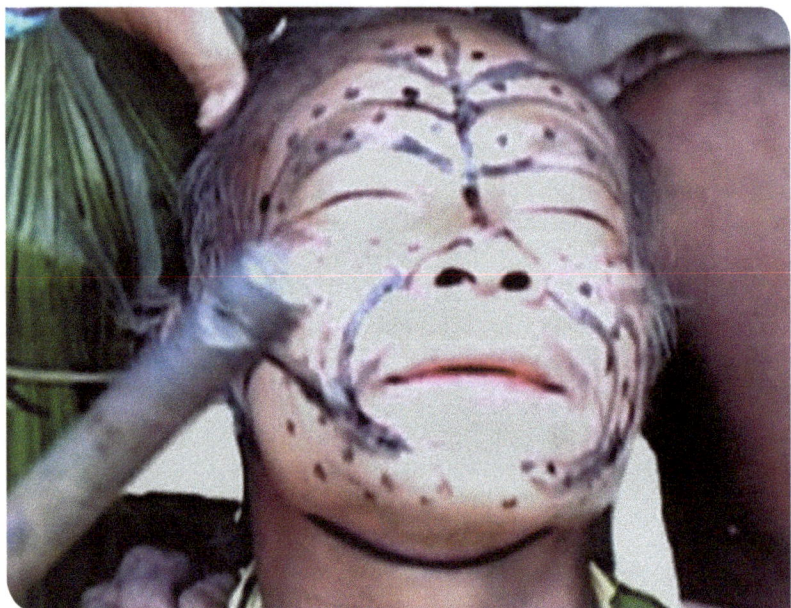

Fig. 1.4: Traditional method of tattooing.
Source: Image courtesy http://www.thebetterindia.com/58170/india-tattoo-tradition-history/.

bearing tissue, which can function as a matrix for the pigment for a life-time. The pigment can be pricked into the skin or rubbed into small cuts in the skin, carried out using a cutting object, with or without wanting to create scar formation in addition to the tattoo. It is believed that prehistoric man cut holes in his skin, charred sticks in the fire, let them cool and then applied the black substance to the wound to create tribal markings.[1] In the Pacific Ocean area, a technique was practiced where the needle was placed at an angle of about 90° on a stick. The stick was hit or hammered with fre-quent blows, so that the pigment placed on the skin was put in the corium in almost the same way as modern tattoo machine. A straight stick with a shape nearly like a drumstick was used as a hammer (Fig. 1.4).

Electric tattoo machines were introduced as a patented tattoo machine in 1891 by the American Samuel F O'Reilly. This machine was powered by a small rotating electric motor. In 1899, the Englishman Alfred Charles developed the tattoo machine that was based on two coils and electromag-netism, which conquered the world, and which is the dominant type today. However, recently improved rotary machines are making a comeback. Tattoo machines were the technical prerequisite for the very large prevalence of tattooing in Europe and other industrialized societies, introduced by sea-farers everywhere, starting in the seaports. Since the 1700s seafarers have been tattooed when they were out in the world on dangerous voyages with sailing ships to faraway lands. It was the seafarers and the opening of the seven seas that brought tattoos to Europe.

TATTOO IN FIELD OF MEDICINE

Tattooing as a form of therapy was perhaps as early as the 4th–5th millennium BC. In 1991 in the Ötztaler Alps in Austria near Innsbruck, a frozen mummy was found, the Iceman—popularly called "Ötzi". The well-preserved mummy had black tattoos in the form of parallel lines that were tattooed into the skin across the large joints, such as the wrist joints, knee joints and foot joints, as well as on the back. It is assumed that the tattoos were medically performed in order to heal joint discomfort.[15-17] The placement of these tattoos on the lines of the spinal cord, behind the knees and ankles suggest the use of the practice as a form of acupuncture therapy. A crude practice of medical tattooing was performed by Galen in 150 CE. He tried to cover leukomatous opacities of the cornea by cauterizing the surface with a heated stilet and applying powdered nutgalls and iron or pulverized pomegranate bark mixed with copper salt.[18]

The Tibetans equated designs called mantra wheels were tattooed on chakra (energy points) on the body to help the bearer of the tattoo achieve physical, emotional and spiritual harmony. Sometimes tattoos were created from medicinal dyes and marked on acupuncture points of the body in an attempt to cure chronic health problems and diseases. Older Maori women tattooed their lips and face to prevent failing vision. Ainu women of Japan tattooed a Goddess on their skin so that the evil spirits that bestowed disease would mistake them for the Goddess and flee in terror. In India, the Lord Hanuman was also tattooed on dislocated shoulders. In mid-1800s, A German physician Pauli used tattooing with mercury sulfide and white lead for the restoration of the natural color to the skin in cases on congenital vascular nevi. Other instances include the cosmetic tattooing with mercury sulfide after plastic lip procedures recommended by Shule in 1850 or the modern method of corneal tattooing put into practice by Louis Von Wecker in the 1870s.[19] Now, medical therapeutic tattooing has been used as a camouflage technique in vitiligo, for breast areola reconstruction after cancer surgery, as camouflage for permanent hair loss after craniofacial surgery, and scars following plastic and reconstructive surgery.[20]

EPIDEMIOLOGY OF TATTOOING

In recent times, tattoos have steadily become more popular, particularly among young people as a means of self-expression or being different, and new social and cultural movements continue to support the popularity of such practices.[21] 10–30% of the adult population of industrialized countries are now tattooed.[22] It has been suggested that there might be an association between risk behaviors and piercing and tattooing practices.[23]

Rising Trends of Tattooing in Adolescence

According to the studies, the prevalence of tattoos in adolescents ranges from 4.5% to 23% and thus "age of adolescence" form first age for tattooing. Boys are three times more likely to get tattoo done than girls. However, recent Harris interactive study 2012 showed that adults aged 30–39 years are most likely to have a tattoo (38%) compared to both those younger (30% of those 25–29 years) and 22% of those 18–24 years.[24] The reasons invoked by youth for tattooing or piercing refer mostly to the expression of individuality (i.e. to feel unique and special), to the confirmation of their personal identity, and to esthetics.[25] A study by S Balci et al. among college going students showed significant association between getting tattoos and the students' risk-taking habits of smoking, taking alcohol, addictive substance use, use of stimulant substances/pills, engaging in extreme sports, carrying sticks/switch blades/gas sprays, engaging in unprotected sex and frequently changing sexual partners. Tattoos are mostly seen on the back, shoulders, arms and legs.[23] A study stated that friends were an important factor in the decision to have tattoos done. Armstrong et al. found that 63% of the students had the intention of getting another piercing and that 64% were thinking of getting another tattoo.[26] Galle et al. reported that 53.6% of the students had their piercings and tattoos done at professional establishments and also that sterile and disposable instruments were used in the procedures in the case of 70.6%. These findings are a positive indication that young people generally contact reliable establishments to get their piercings and tattoos.[27] Under the circumstances, it is imperative that young people receive education about the risks of piercing and tattooing and that the importance of having these performed by professionally trained people under sterile conditions is impressed upon them. Despite the increasing number of tattooed individuals, there are currently few requirements, little legislation and few criteria for the safety of tattoos.

TATTOOING AND BEHAVIORAL RISK

Given growth in popularity of tattoos, the prevalence and characteristics of those who have been tattooed have changed in the past decade. Professional tattooers with salons are on rise and amateur tattooing and self-tattooing are on decrease in urban areas. Uniqueness and gender seem to be motivating factors in tattoo procurement. In one study involving career-oriented women with tattoos, many of whom were counselors, nurses, physicians, lawyers, and business managers, deliberate decision making and self-controlled body site placement were described as assistive for their tattoo satisfaction. The tattoos symbolized individuality and identity, projecting both femininity and personal strength.[28]

Historically, tattooing has been associated with gang-related activities, drug use, prisoners and also underlying psychopathology. Tattoos are now regularly seen on celebrities, athletes, and middle-class young people. Tattooing is also viewed as a form of deviant behavior. Some studies have shown an increased prevalence of tattoos in young individuals attempting suicide.[29] Among adolescents, tattooing has been associated with drug, and alcohol use, increased levels of sexual activity, suicide ideation, and illegal/violent behavior. A study using random digit dialing in the United States in 2004 survey 24% respondents had tattoos, with those who were younger, lower paid, had spent time in prison, used alcohol or drugs, and had achieved lower levels of education reporting the highest levels of tattooing.[30]

EPIDEMIOLOGY OF TATTOO-RELATED DISEASE TRANSMISSION

One of the earliest sources linking disease transmission to the practice of tattooing can be found in MF Hutin's "Recherches sur les Tatouages", published in 1853. He relates the case of a tattooed soldier who suffered from syphilis due to misdeed of tattooist who remoistened dried ink with his saliva infected with *Spirochaetaceae*.[31] After Hutin, and until the end of the century, only five cases of primary syphilis, from 1900 onwards there is decrease in trend of cases reported probably due to shift in the professional practices and standards of tattooists.[32] Similarly, the trend from syphilis and tuberculosis in the late 19th and early 20th centuries shifted to hepatitis from around the 1950s right up until 1980, and HIV in the 1980s And '90s. Tattooing and body piercing can be possible vectors for the transmission of blood-borne diseases such as hepatitis B, hepatitis C or HIV. A 1999 United Kingdom survey of family practitioners showed that 95% of them have seen patients with complications resulting from a piercing.[33]

A study of 31 female patients with leprosy lesions starting over tattoo marks was reported from a leprosy endemic area from India. In most cases, improper use of hygiene regimens, particularly contaminated needles are causal, but sometimes, contaminated pigments are implicated. Severe systemic mycoses can be transmitted rarely by tattooing.[20]

CONCLUSION

Tattoos have been around for centuries. As a form of identity, they have existed across cultures and geographies. They reflect time and society, and change as they change. The concept of tattooing has extended its arms even in medicinal healing science. Its knowledge has paved way through centuries and has survived through modern era with varied application. As the trend for getting tattoo is increasing, so is the awareness about professional tattooing and tattoo-related complications. Nowadays, the incidence of tattoo removal has also been more common.

REFERENCES

1. Dorfer L, Moser M, Bahr F, et al. A medical report from the Stone Age? Lancet. 1999;354:1023-5.
2. Wolfa AD, Robitailleb B, Krutakc L, et al. The World's Oldest Tattoos. J Archaeol Sci: Reports. 2016. [online] Available at http://www.sciencedirect.com/science/article/pii/S2352409X15301772. [Accessed April, 2017].
3. Schmid S. Tattoos—An historical essay. Travel Med Infect Dis. 2013;11:444-7.
4. Hooker JD. Captain Cook's journal during his first voyage round the world made in H.M. Bark "Endeavour" 1768-71. Nature. 1893;1235(48):195-6.
5. Graudenz K, Greve B, Raulin C. Diffused traumatic dirt and decorative tattooing: Removal by Q-switched lasers. Hautarzt. 2003;54:756-9.
6. Isaacs D. Tattoos. J Paediatr Child Health. 2012;48(12):1051-2.
7. Krutak L. Spiritual skin: magical tattoos and scarification. Germany: Edition Reuss; 2013.
8. The Bible. (2015). Leviticus, 19:28. [online] Available at http://da.bibelsite.com/leviticus/19-28.htm. [Accessed April, 2017].
9. Poysden M, Bratt M. A History of Japanese Body Suit Tattooing. Amsterdam: KIT Publishers; 2006.
10. Taschen's 1000 Biker Tattoos. (2014). [online] Available at http://www.print-mytattoo.com/members/ebooks/The%20Tattoo%20E-Book.pdf. [Accessed April, 2017]. [Accessed April, 2017].
11. Haq S. The Skin and the Ink: Tracing the Boundaries of Tattoo Art in India. [online] Available at http://network.icom.museum/fileadmin/user_upload/minisites/cidoc/BoardMeetings/Sarah_Haq.pdf [Accessed April, 2017].
12. Mohanta BK. Tattoo And Tribal Identity: A case of the Baiga tribe of Central India. Asian Mirror—International Journal of Research, Volume II, Issue II, May-2015;80-7.
13. de Groot AC. Side-effects of henna and semi-permanent "black henna" tattoos: a full review. Contact Dermatitis. 2013;69:1-25.
14. Oanță A, Irimie M, Brănișteanu DE, et al. Tattoos— History and Actuality. Bulletin of the Transilvania University of Brașov Series VI: Medical Sciences. 2014;7(56):1-8.
15. Krutak L. Spiritual skin: magical tattoos and scarification. Germany: Edition Reuss, 2013.
16. Sulzenbacher G. The glacier mummy (Discovering the Neolithic Age with the Iceman). Folio. Vienna-Bolzano and South Tyrol of Archeology; 2006.
17. Zieglar SL. Multicolor tattooing of the cornea. Trans Am Ophthalmol Soc. 1922;20:71-87.
18. Turell R, Marino AW. Technic of tattooing with mercury sulfide for pruritus ani. Ann Surg. 1942;115:126-30.

19. Von Wecker L. Das Tätowiren der Hornhaut. Arch Augenheilkunde. 1872;2:84-7.
20. Khunger N, Molpariya A, Khunger A. Complications of Tattoos and Tattoo Removal: Stop and Think Before you ink. J Cutan Aesthetic Surg. 2015;8(1):30-6.
21. Huxley C, Grogan S. Tattooing, piercing, healthy behaviours and health value. J Health Psychol. 2005;10:831-41.
22. Laumann AE. History and epidemiology of tattoos and piercings. Legislation in the United States. In: De Cuyper C, Perez-Cotapos ML (Eds). Dermatologic complications with body art. Berlin-Heidelberg: Springer-Verlag; 2010. pp. 1-11.
23. Oliveria SM, Matos MA, Martins R, et al. Tattooing and body piercing as lifestyle indicator of risk behaviors in Brazilian adolescents. Eur J Epidemiol. 2006;21:559-60.
24. Aiyedun V, Ncube F. Literature review on the epidemiology of tattooing and its complications. V0.7. Health Protection Agency, Colindale
25. Deschesnes M, Demers S, Finès P. Prevalence and Characteristics of Body Piercing and Tattooing Among High School Students. Canadian J Pub Health. 2006;97(4):325-9.
26. Armstrong ML, Roberts AE, Owen DC, et al. Contemporary college students and body piercing. J Adolesc Health. 2004;35:58-61.
27. Gallè F, Mancusi C, Di Onofrio V, et al. Awareness of health risks related to body art practices among youth in Naples, Italy: a descriptive convenience sample study. BMC Public Health. 2011;11:625
28. Armstrong ML. Career-oriented women with tattoos. Image J Nurs Sch. 1991; 23(4):215-20.
29. Stephens MB. Behavioral Risks Associated With Tattooing. Clin Res Methods Fam Med. 2003;35(1):52-4.
30. Laumann AE, Derick AJ. Tattoos and body piercings in the United States: A national data set. J Am Acad Dermatol. 2006;55:413-21.
31. Gemma Angel. Atavistic marks and risky Practices: the tattoo in medical-legal debate 1850-1950. In: Reinarz J, Siena K (Eds). A Medical History of Skin: Scratching the Surface. London: Pickering Chatto; 2013. pp. 165-79.
32. Rickman LS. Infectious Complications of Tattoos. Clin Infect Dis. 1994;18(4):612-3.
33. AEGiS. Piercing problems for 'one in five'. BBC News. (2002). [online] Available at http://www.aegis.com/news/bbc/2002/BB020104.html. [Accessed April, 2017].

Chapter 2

Types of Tattoos

Shashikumar BM

INTRODUCTION

Tattooing is a very old practice which involves insertion of ink pigment of the desired color into the dermis. It is prevailing among most of the societies worldwide and is becoming increasingly common in the developing countries.[1] Tattoos can broadly be divided into permanent or temporary.[2] Permanent tattooing is the insertion of dye/pigment into the deep dermis using needles and intended to be permanent, whereas temporary tattoos are composed mainly of henna, which is painted on skin surface rather than inserting deep into the skin. It is intended to wear off with epidermal turnover.

PERMANENT TATTOOS

These are practiced worldwide and across all cultures. These are broadly classified as:[2,3]
- Decorative tattoos
- Medical/reconstructive tattoos
- Traumatic tattoos.

Decorative Tattoos

Decorative tattoos are the most common type and the largest group of permanent tattoos. It can be classifed in many ways, though no stringent classifcation exists. Decorative tattoos can be classifed depending on the ways of tattooing and material used or depending on design and site (Table 2.1).

Table 2.1: Types of decorative tattoo.[3,4]

Depending on the ways of tattooing and material used	Depending on design and site
• Amateur tattoo • Professional tattoo	• Cosmetic tattoos • Emblem/tribal/group tattoos • Identification tattoos • Extensive tattoos • Impulse tattoos • Intimate and mucous membrane tattoos • Effect tattoos

Professional Tattoos

Professional tattoos have become very popular these days, especially among youngsters. Many youngsters are choosing tattooing as their career. In Indian set-up, there are no set rules, educational norms or authorization requirements to designate artists as professionals. But, presence of artisanal experience, an esthetic qualification, and insight into the use of ink and equipment and knowledge about medical conditions, especially regarding infectious diseases, asepsis and hygiene should be mandate for a professional tattoo artist.[3,4]

A tattoo machine is used to deposit the pigment into the deeper layer of the dermis in a professional way in a modern esthetic set-up, taking hygiene into consideration. There are two main varieties of tattoo machines, whose principle is almost the same: (1) rotary tattoo machines, and (2) coil tattoo machines (Figs. 2.1A and B).[5] Both defer in weight, noise and versatility but selection of which depends on the artist's ease and choice.

1. *Rotary tattoo machines:* It consists of small motor that moves the attached tattoo needles up and down in a smooth, almost cyclical pattern. Rotary tattoo machines move needles in and out of the skin more fluidly and evenly.
2. *Coil tattoo machines:* It is a traditional machine that works on electromagnetic current passed through a pair of coils to trigger a draw and release of the machine's armature bar. It has a very hammer-like effect, with the release of the springs causing the armature bar to essentially tap the attached tattoo needles into the skin.

Also, tattoo ink used by artists differs in many aspects. Though these inks falls under the purview of Food and Drug Administration as cosmetic color additives, their ingredients are usually kept secret by many companies. A tattoo ink basically consists of two components: (1) pigment and (2) vehicle. Tattoo pigment is the most important component, consisting of

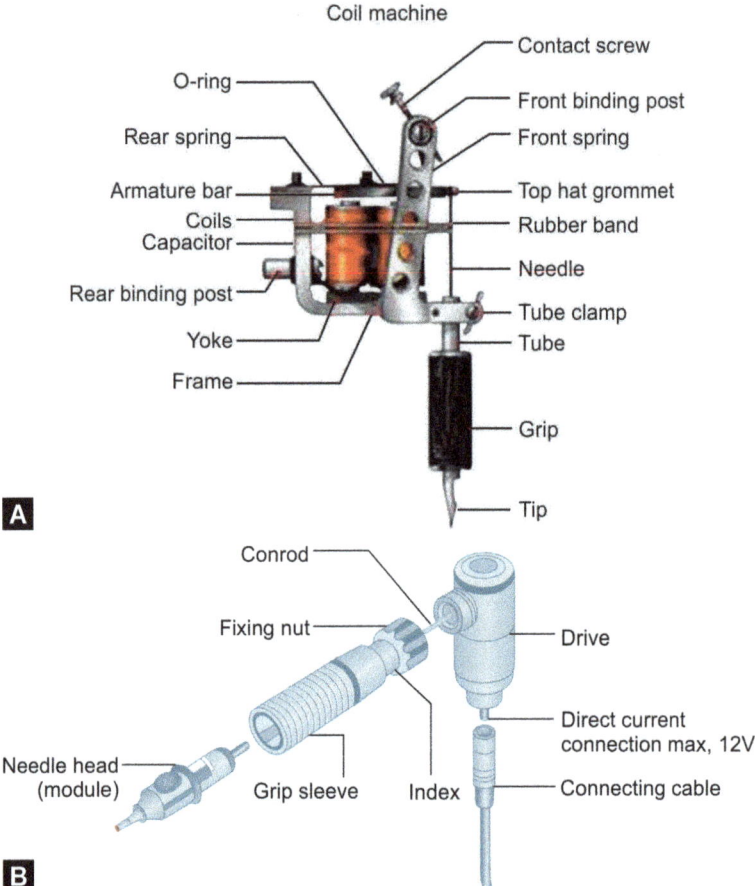

Figs. 2.1A and B: Types of tattoo machine: rotary tattoo machines and coil tattoo machines.

heavy metals, metal oxides or organic dyes whereas vehicle is solvent which entraps, encases, incorporates, complexes, encapsulates, or is otherwise associated with the pigment to form pigment/vehicle complexes that helps to retain the pigment in the tissue. Whatever may be the ingredients, tattoo ink should be inert, nonallergic, safe and nontoxic.[3]

Basic skills of tattooing: Tattooing is an art which is mastered with practice and fashion. Following are the basic aspects considered while tattooing:

• *Design:* Basic step in tattooing is the selection of suitable design. It can be a text, a symbol, an ornament or a figure. Many a times templates are available on which an artist works.

• *Lining:* It is the technique used to create a basic shape of the intended design over the skin surface. Usually dark colors are used for lining. Lining tends to be done with a single pass, with short tapering needles arranged in circular pattern.

- *Coloring:* It refers to filling the designed areas with appropriate color. Filling is done with long needles and goes with multiple passes.
- *Shading:* It can be created by using different length of needle and pressure. Also, its different shading can be done by mixing the dye with lighter color or with diluting the dye.

Amateur Tattoos

It is done by untrained artists. Most commonly performed in rural places and in fair on roadside or makeshift parlor (Figs. 2.2 and 2.3). It is done using homemade tattoo machine (Fig. 2.4), needle or thrones. Common substances used are charcoal, pen ink, soot, organic dye or fabric dyes. Amateur tattoos are of single color, lighter in color and applied more superficially. Thus removal is easier than professional tattoo. Also, depth of tattooing is not uniform in amateur tattoos.

Cosmetic Tattoos

They are also known as permanent makeup. Colors similar to makeup are used to color, expand or line the border of lips by tattooing. Similarly cosmetic tattoos are used as permanent eyeliner and also to mark or create hanging eyebrows. Bindi tattoo is a type of cosmetic tattoo. Tittoing is a type of cosmetic tattooing done to augment the color of nipples and areola. Tatteeth is the tattooing of teeth and tooth crowns. Special tattoo machines

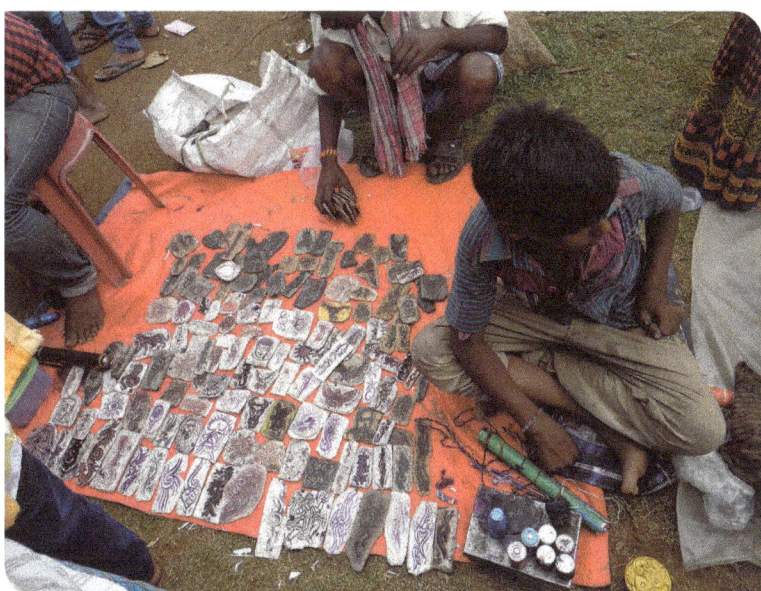

Fig. 2.2: Make shift tattoo in fair.

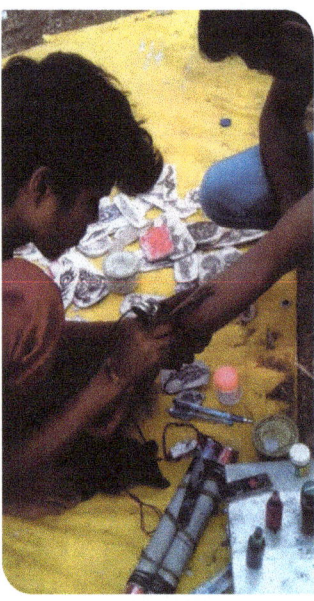

Fig. 2.3: Tattooing at the fair in an unsterile environment.

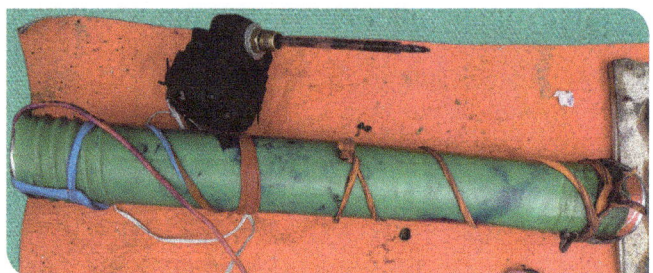

Fig. 2.4: Homemade tattoo machine.

with thin needles are used for this purpose. Common colors used are brown, pink, red and black. Semipermanent inks are also available in the market.

Emblem/Group/Tribal Tattoos

Emblem tattoo signifies individual affiliation to an organization. Military tattoo, sailors tattoo among navy officers are some examples. Similarly individual's affiliation to certain group is depicted through gang's symbol. Japanese gang tattoos, Biker's tattoo, Hispanic and Mexican gang tattoos are popular group tattoos. Tribal tattoos were present since centuries and practiced widely across the world but were widespread among general population in 19th century. Other names for tribal tattoos are magic or ethnic tattoos. Unique facial tattoo among Maoris of New Zealand are well-known.

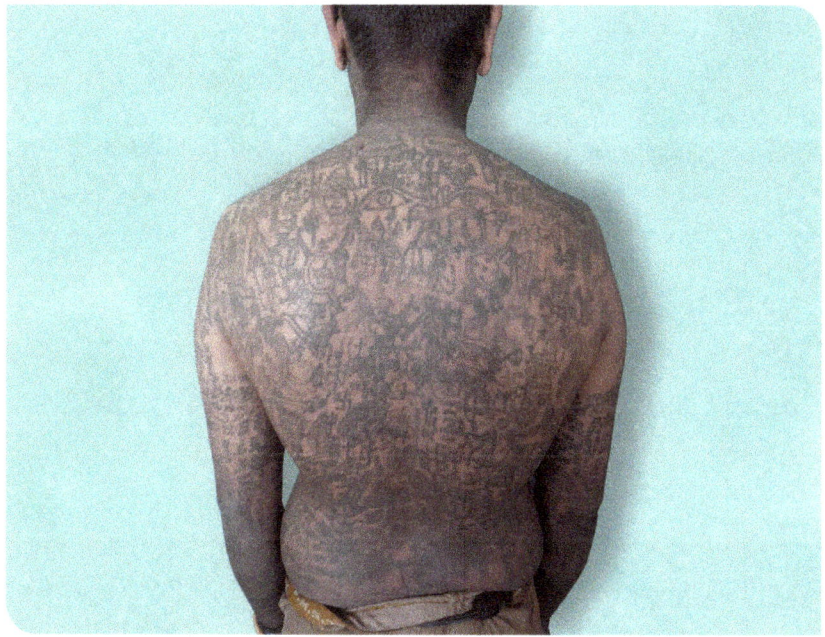

Fig. 2.5: Extensive tattoo in a destitute.

Identification Tattoos

Individual's personnel details like name, date of birth or similar data are engraved on the skin. Commonly employed in concentration camp of Nazi's, where inmates were tattooed with identification numbers and special symbols. It is also worn by seafarers, soldiers and civilians. Alzheimer's patients were carved with their name on the forearm for easy identification. Similarly many people wore tattoo of their blood group to enable transfusion in emergency situation. During World War II, members of the Nazi Waffen-SS troop wore blood group tattoos for identification.

Extensive Tattoos

Tattoos covering more than 80% body surface are known as extensive tattoos (Fig. 2.5). People with extensive tattoos are more prone for deviant behavior especially people with asymmetrical, noncorrelative tattoo over the body.

Impulse Tattoos

Decision to get tattooed is taken in a hurry or sudden impulse of an otherwise normal person. Many a time it may be due to impaired decision-making due to inebriation, or drugs or medicine, which affects the psyche and judgment. These are the known seekers for tattoo removal.

Intimate and Mucous Membrane Tattoos

Intimate tattoos are provocative and respire erotic mood. Women make intimate tattoos on their body more often than men. Preferred areas for tattooing are genital area, inner thighs, buttocks, breasts and lower back. Risk and complications are more and also with years, body shape may change, making tattoo ugly or irrelevant. Mucosal tattoos are placed in oral cavity, genital mucosa and sclera of eye.

Effect Tattoos

Glow in the dark tattoo is a new trend in the market and they contain phosphorus which fluorescence in the dark. Three-dimensional tattoo images have grown more common over the past few years and contain special implants in addition to tattoo pigment.

Newer Tattoos[6,7]

- *Animated tattoos:* It contains programmable subcutaneous visible implant (PSVI), a liquid crystal display (LCD) screen with preprogrammed images implanted under the skin along with tattoo pigment above. Images can be reprogrammed. Their medical uses are being explored.
- *Random tattoos:* QR code in impregnated on skin similar to tattooing. Scanning the QR code can fetch the information.
- *Eye color tattoos:* Dye is injected into the iris to change the ethnical color of the eye. Similar it can be injected into the sclera. But corneal tattoo is a type of tattooing done for corneal opacities.
- *Electronic tattoos:* It is also known as emotion tattoos. It is an invisible tattoo which appears on the surface of the skin and travel across the body, following the person's touch. It is meant for those who want to keep their tattoos a secret.

Medical Reconstructive Tattoos[8-10]

Tattooing is extensively used in the medical field earlier in the form of medical alert tattooing, cosmetic tattooing, esthetic or reconstructive tattoos (Table 2.2). Tattoo machine and needles used are similar to professional tattoos (Figs. 2.6A and B). Medical alert tattooing includes information about one's blood group or medical condition like penicillin or other drug allergies, epilepsy, diabetic, etc. which are tattooed over visible parts like forearm. Reconstructive tattooing of breast nipples and the surrounding areola are carried out after breast cancer surgery.

Table 2.2: Medical use of tattooing.

Medical alert	Cosmetic tattooing
• Specific health conditions like epilepsy • Penicillin and other drug allergy • Blood group • Do not resuscitate (DNR) directives	• Permanent eye lining, lip coloring, etc. • Eye color tattooing
Reconstructive tattoo	Micropigmentation
• Postsurgery breast and nipple reconstruction • Camouflage for permanent hair loss after craniofacial surgery • Scars following plastic and reconstructive surgery	• Port-wine stains, nevus flammeus, capillary hemangiomas • Vitiligo, leucoderma • Alopecia areata, androgenetic alopecia • Syringomata other benign appendageal tumors

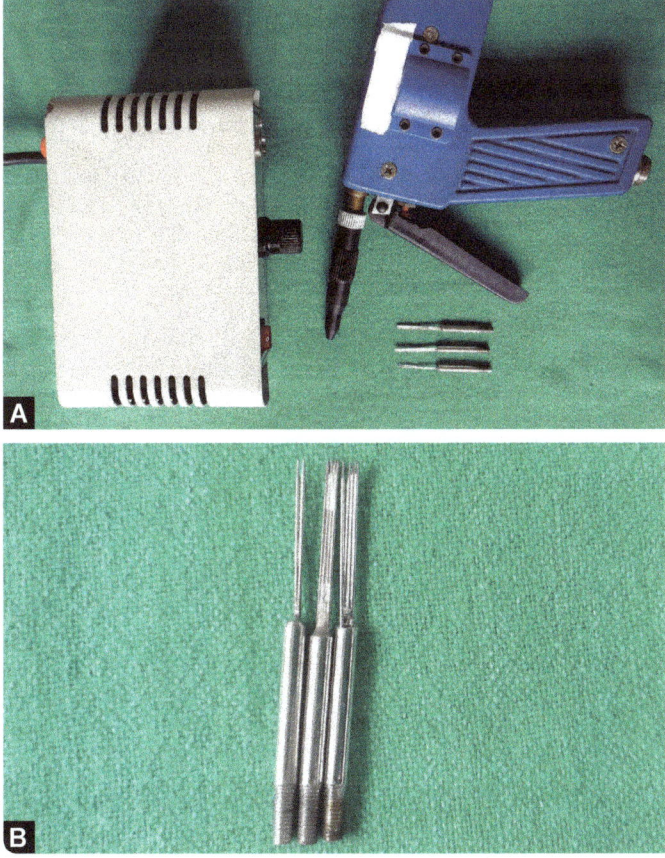

Figs. 2.6A and B: Tattoo machine used for micropigmentation. Insert showing various types of needles used.

In dermatology, esthetic tattooing of scalp known as micropigmentation is done to create the illusion of hair over scalp in hair loss conditions. Also, it is done in scarring alopecia or nonresponding alopecia areata. Tattooing is done in vitiligo and other leucoderma as cosmetic camouflage. Details are given in Chapter 5.

Traumatic Tattoos

It is due to abrasion or laceration following road traffic accident or explosive injuries, leading to deposition of particles in skin layers giving rise to blue or black color. Graphite from pencil may be deposited following injury especially in children.

TEMPORARY TATTOOS

In contrast to permanent tattoos, designs are painted on the surface of the skin in temporary tattoos which will lasts for weeks to months. Here, color will binds with skin surface which is removed over few weeks with the spontaneous renewal of the epidermis and exfoliation. Many types of temporary tattoos are described but henna is the most ancient and widely used temporary tattoo.

Types

- Henna
- Airbrush tattoos
- Decal-style temporary tattoos
- Metallic jewelry tattoos.

Henna

Henna is a flowering plant, *Lawsonia inermis* and also refers to dye derived from the leaves of the same plant. *Lawsonia* is the chemical present in the dye which stains the skin. It gives reddish-brown color to skin, hair and nail. It lasts for few weeks.

Airbrush Tattoos

Airbrush is used to create the desired design using a stencil. It lasts for short duration. It is removed with rubbing alcohol or baby oil. Airbrush temporary tans are a common form of airbrush tattoos wherein dihydroxyacetone (DHA) which reacts with the amino acids in the outer layer of the skin is used to create a tanned appearance.

Decal-style Temporary Tattoos

Decal is a short form of word "decalcomania". A design embedded on a paper is transferred by pressing it on the skin surface. It is very popular among children.

Metallic Jewelry Tattoos

It is similar to decal tattoo, but gold or silver foil is used to press on the skin. Both last for a week.

SEMIPERMANENT TATTOOS

Freedom-2 LLC is new tattoo which is applied similar to permanent tattooing but ink can be removed with just a single laser treatment.

CONCLUSION

There are many types of tattoos classified in different ways. Tattooing as an art, emerging with many newer tools and designs, medical uses of which is being explored.

REFERENCES

1. Shashikumar BM, Harish MR, Shwetha B, et al. Hypersensitive reaction to tattoos: a growing menace in rural India. Indian J Dermatol. Forthcoming 2017.
2. Khunger N, Molpariya A, Khunger A. Complications of Tattoos and Tattoo Removal: Stop and Think Before you ink. J Cutan Aesthet Surg. 2015;8(1):30-6.
3. Serup J, Harrit N, Linnet JT, et al. Tattoos – Health, Risks and Culture. With an introduction to the "seamless prevention" strategy. Copenhagen: The Council on Health and Disease Prevention. 2015;1-156.
4. Ho SG, Goh CL. Laser tattoo removal: a clinical update. J Cutan Aesthet Surg. 2015;8(1):9-15.
5. Painful Pleasures. (2014). Coil vs. Rotary Tattoo Machines. [online] Available from info.painfulpleasures.com/help-center/information-center/coil-vs-rotary-tattoo-machines. [Accessed April, 2017].
6. Welcome to Tattooing 101.com. (2017). The Different Styles and Techniques of Tattooing. [online] Available from tattooing101.com/the-different-styles-and-techniques-of-tattooing. [Accessed April, 2017].
7. Taylor C. (2017). Ink Innovation for the Information Age The Tattoo Revolution. [online] Available from dishmag.com/issue174/lifestyle/15376/awesome-tattoo-revolution. [Accessed April, 2017].
8. Epstein E. Therapeutic tattooing. In: Epstein E (Ed). Skin Surgery, 2nd edition. Philadelphia: Lea & Febiger; 1962. pp. 308-15.
9. Conway H. Tattooing of nevus flammeus for permanent camouflage. J Am Med Assoc. 1953;152(8):666-9.
10. Garg G, Thami GP. Micropigmentation: tattooing for medical purposes. Dermatol Surg. 2005;31(8 Pt 1):928-31.

Chapter 3

Composition of Tattoo

Savitha AS

INTRODUCTION

The act of tattooing has been practised since many centuries. The tattooing process involves inserting ink pigment of the desired color into the dermal layer of the skin.

Products used for tattooing are a mixture of chemicals that absorb visible light, the actual colorants, and a large spectrum of auxiliary ingredients (Table 3.1).

The coloring agents used in tattoos are mainly of two subgroups:
1. *The pigments*: Metallic salts (oxides, sulfides, and selenides) or organic molecules of different origin.
2. *The dyes*: Mostly organic molecules.

Table 3.1: Constituents of tattoo.	
Colorant	Pigment
	Dye
Auxiliary ingredients	*Vehicle*: water Solvent Additives: • *Wetting agents*: Glycerin, ethylene glycol • *Preservatives*: Witch hazel • *Stabilizer* • *Thickeners*: Glycerin • *pH regulators*
Impurities from the production process	

PREPARATION OF TATTOO INK

Tattoo ink is a suspension of pigment particles in a solution of water, glycerin, and alcohol (mostly ethanol or isopropanol). Pigments are tiny, insoluble solid particles and are not affected by the medium in which they are incorporated. The structure of a pigment will not alter during the coloring process. The size of the microcrystalline particles will define the color of the end product. To prepare tattoo ink, pure pigment powder or a predispersed paste is used.

Predispersed paste is a mixture of pure pigment powder and acrylonitrile butadiene styrene (ABS) which is plastic processed to microparticles and wetted to obtain a paste, which is much easier to handle; the amount of plastic can be adapted to obtain different shades. In order to make a stable suspension the polar properties of the pigments can be modified by using *additives*; this process is called *wetting*.[1] In contrast to pigments, dyes are soluble either in water or in some organic nonpolar solvent. The dyes consist of a stabilizer (mostly barium sulfate) with a colored surface (e.g. acid azo dye). For the traditional tattooing purposes, mostly pigments are used because they offer a high light stability and are chemically resistant, especially the metallic salts. They remain unchanged in contrast to the "stabilized" dyes. Dyes have a tendency to fade over time, an advantage in the indication of permanent make up (semipermanent), while pigments will persist unaffected and permanent, as is the objective in ornamental tattoos.

EVOLUTION OF COLORANTS

In ancient times, materials used for tattooing consisted minerals, plant extracts, soot, carbon, and ochre; the same products are still used nowadays in ethnic tattoos. Indian ink, also called Chinese ink, has been used since at least the fourth century BC. In India, the carbon black from which the Indian ink is produced was obtained by burning bones, tar, pitch, lampblack, and other substances. Carbon black is a powder that mainly comprises amorphous particles of carbon with diameters of a few tenths of a nanometer.[2] Colorants mentioned in the literature used for traditional tattooing include mineral pigments and metallic oxides/hydroxides/sulfides/aluminates such as chrome for green, cobalt and indigo for blue, cadmium sulfide for yellow, and mercury sulfide or cinnabar for red. Soot derivatives and carbon pigments (graphite) are still used nowadays for black inks.

During the 1980s, complex organic colorants gained popularity; nowadays, 80% of the pigments are synthetic organic molecules mostly azo pigments and polycyclic compounds.[3] In the category of organic pigments, common are azo dyes (orange, brown, yellow, and red) and other polycyclic

Table 3.2: Pigments used in tattoo.

Color	Metals	Organic	Other
Black	-	-	Charcoal, carbon
Brown	Ferric oxide, cadmium sulfide	-	-
White	Lead carbonate, zinc oxide, titanium dioxide	-	-
Violet	-	Azo dyes	Manganese
Purple/lilac	-		Manganese oxide
Flesh	Ferric oxide	-	-
Green	Chromium oxide (casalic green), hydrous chromium oxides (Guignets green), chromium sesquioxide (Viridian)	Chlorinated copper (phthalocyanine)	-
Red	Mercury sulfide (cinnabar), cadmium selenide	Azo dyes	Sienna, brazilin, carmine cochinilla red, santalin
Yellow	Cadmium sulfide	Azo dyes	-
Blue	Cobalt	Copper (phthalocyanine)	Indigo

amines, dioxazine, phthalocyanine, quinacridone, and arylide. In many tattoo inks, titanium dioxide is used as a lightener; titanium dioxide however has a risk for paradoxical darkening when treated with laser.[4]

Natural pigments being used nowadays are colorant extractions from trees, flowers and roots such as curcumine (Curcuma), brazilin (Brazil wood = natural red 24), and santalin (red sandalwood = natural red 22/23) (Tables 3.2 and 3.3).

In recent years, heavy metals, mercury (cinnabar) and cadmium responsible for allergic reactions in red and yellow tattoos have been replaced by synthetic molecules.[5]

OTHER INGREDIENTS

To obtain a stable tattoo ink, additives and a carrier medium are needed. Additives with a thickening effect and surface-active chemicals needed to change the polar properties of the pigments are used in order obtain a homogenous solution. These additives can help to make the ink stick to the tattooing needle. Because organic material and water are subject to bacterial and fungal contamination, preservatives like benzoic acid are often added to the tattooing products. Even local anesthetics have also been

Table 3.3: Types of pigments.

Mineral pigments		
• Iron oxides	*Heavy metals*: Mercury, cadmium, zinc, lead, chromium	
	Others: Titanium	
Organic pigments		
• Azo compounds	Light stable, cheap and easy to produce, insoluble in water, but often soluble in alcohol or solvents Azo compounds are fragile and under influence of high energetic radiation and heat aromatic amines can be created. Azo compounds are mostly yellow, orange, red, magenta or purple	
• Phthalocyanine compounds	Very stable and safe, only blue and green, insoluble in water and most solvents	

mixed.[6] The carrier usually consists of water, alcohol, and glycerin. Common solvents that function as carriers are ethanol or isopropanol. Popular carrier components include hamamelis extract, propylene glycol, and glycerol. Listerine and vodka are often used for thinning of traditional tattoo inks.[1]

Unsafe substances recovered from tattoo inks are methanol, ethylene glycol, aldehydes (glutaraldehyde), detergents, and benzoates.

TATTOO PIGMENTS ROUTE THROUGH THE SKIN AND BODY

Tattooing injects the ink with thousands of vertical needle pricks into the dermis. This is carried out by first dipping a needled tattoo instrument into the colored ink before applying to the skin. The oscillating ink-coated needle punctures the skin in the range of 100 times per second, depositing the ink pigments 1.5–2 mm below the skin surface. Thus, the needle penetrates the skin through the epidermis and into the papillary layer of the dermis, where the ink particles accumulate. As with any type of trauma to the dermis, the first response of the body is to stop the resultant bleeding to form a clot. Then there is edema, followed by a migration of neutrophils and macrophages in order to phagocytose foreign substance. In the initial few days after tattooing, some of the tattoo color will be rejected by the skin together with desquamated scabs and dead skin cells, or seep into the bandaging. Soluble substances in the ink and the vehicle in the form of water and isopropanol will probably distribute itself locally in the tissue and move into the bloodstream within a short period of time. The poorly soluble particles, such as the pigment particles will also move locally in the tissue and toward the vessels, so that the particles have a certain possibility to move out of the skin and through the lymph vessels to the regional lymph nodes in the armpits or groin.[7] The regional lymph nodes are the most important first pass organ before the route to the bloodstream. The wounded papillary dermis is then repaired through the action of fibroblasts, ultimately laying down scar tissue. Over long periods of time the tattoo ink particles can be found to gradually move to the deeper dermis which gives the tattoo a faded and blurred appearance. In a studies with mice, nanoparticles can, in addition to being in the tattooed skin and the regional lymph nodes, be shown in organs such as the liver and the spleen as soon as 24 hours later.[8]

Toxicity of Tattoo Pigments

In a report by Baeumler et al. it was found that some of the azo-type colorants contained aromatic amines as impurities, classified as carcinogens.[6] Results from the study revealed that of the 52 organic colorants identified in the marketplace 17% contained a carcinogenic aromatic amine. It was shown that in particular *3,3'-dichlorobenzidine* seems to be the molecule that can possibly be released from the azo-colorants used for tattooing.[9] The following molecules have been identified: *o-anisidine, 4-chloro-o-toluidine, 3,3-dichlorobenzidine, o-toluidine, 2,4-diaminotoluene, which have carcinogenic potential.*[1]

Timko et al. performed an in vitro quantitative chemical analysis of tattoo pigments with the objective to test the accuracy and completeness of information supplied by tattoo ink manufacturers and to perform an elemental assay of tattoo pigments. As a result of this study, the most commonly identified elements were aluminum (87%), oxygen (73%), titanium (67%), and carbon (67% of the pigments).[10]

Although inks are injected into the human body, tattoo inks usually fulfill no pharmaceutical requirements and contain a long list of admixtures and impurities. Black tattoo inks are frequently neither analyzed nor controlled prior to use. Their manufacturing process is based on soot, and so they contain toxic, mutagenic or carcinogenic compounds such as carbon black and polycyclic aromatic hydrocarbons (PAHs) or phenol. PAHs can absorb ultraviolet (UV) radiation and generate cytotoxic singlet oxygen, which might affect skin integrity.[11] A recent Danish study found pathogenic bacteria in 10% of the tattoo ink that was studied.[12]

Photodecomposition products of tattoo pigments could potentially have toxic properties.[13] The effect of natural sunlight on tattoo pigments was also studied by Engel et al. and the presence of primary decomposition products with carcinogenic properties was also demonstrated.[7] When treated with laser there is even an increased risk because carcinogenic decomposition products are released due to the treatment.[14] Until now, the malignancies reported in tattooed individuals have been considered as coincidental, but large epidemiologic studies are needed to prove a relationship between tattooing and cancer. It is unclear whether considerable change in the composition of tattoo products in the last decades, switching more and more to organic azo compounds, will lead to an increase in malignancies.

It is questionable if the exposure to the carcinogens released from tattoos could have an influence that could be comparable to, for example, the exposure to tobacco smoke on the lungs or to sunlight on the skin, an interesting subject for epidemiologists.[15]

RECENT DEVELOPMENTS

The concept of easy removable tattoo inks has been a challenge for the tattoo industry and for researchers involved in laser therapy.[16] Tattoo inks are being developed through the particle encapsulation (P2) and enhancement platform (P2E) a new microbead version of tattoo inks. The removable tattoo ink consists of nanosize pigment particles enclosed in polymer-coated beads of about 1 μm diameter. These microbeads are stored in the dermal macrophage. The polymer beads contain a dopant that absorbs light of a specific wavelength and explode when they are treated with corresponding laser light independent of the color inside the bead. The liberated pigment particles are small enough to be eliminated from the skin. According to the information, the scientists have perfected the dissolution of the pigment so that when treated with laser the tattoo will be gone with fewer treatments.[17]

Temporary Tattoos

The natural source of henna is the plant *Lawsonia inermis*, which is part of the family Lythraceae. The name is derived from Isaac Lawson, assistant of the famous botanist Linnaeus.[18] When applied to the skin, hair, or nails, the pigment lawsone (2-hydroxy-1,4- naphthoquinone; CI 75480; Natural Orange 6), which is present at a concentration of <2% in henna leaves and natural henna preparations, interacts with the keratin therein to give them a reddish-brown ("rust-red") color; therefore, a frequently used synonym is "red henna". At events such as wedding parties, public celebrations, and religious ceremonies, henna is applied to the skin of the hands and feet. The product used is a thick mixture of the dried and powdered plant with water or oil. The paste or liquid is applied with a stick, brush or cotton swab or directly from a syringe, or cone-shaped container onto the skin; it can dry for 20–30 minutes and/or be covered with an occlusive dressing or plastic sheet to enhance penetration in the skin. The dried paste is then removed to reveal an orange stain, which will darken over the next 2–4 days. A temporary henna tattoo should last for approximately 2–6 weeks, until the outer layer of the skin exfoliates, depending on skin type, the area of application, sun exposure, and other factors such as bathing and activity level.[19]

Although natural henna has a very low allergic potential, an increase of reports of allergic reactions to temporary henna tattoos was observed in the last decades due to the use of new mixtures. The structure and redox potential of lawsone (2-hydroxy-1,4-naphthoquinone) are similar to those of 1,4-naphthoquinone, a metabolite of naphthalene and a potent oxidant of glucose-6-phosphate dehydrogenase (G6PD)-deficient cells. Topical application of henna may therefore cause life-threatening hemolysis in children with G6PD deficiency.[20]

Natural henna gives a red color and is known as "red henna". Coffee, black tea, a variety of plant extracts, lime juice and even urine of animals have been used since ages to obtain darker colors. More recently, the addition of other coloring agents creates a larger variety of colors. Temporary black henna tattoo (also sometimes called skin painting or pseudo-tattooing), has become fashionable, ever since the Spice Girls decorated themselves with these body designs. Black henna (sometimes also termed blue henna) is the combination of red henna and para-phenylenediamine (PPD). No natural black henna exists. Some of these "henna" preparations do not even contain red henna at all. PPD is added to henna to:

- Accelerate the dyeing and drying process (to only 30 minutes)
- To strengthen and darken the color
- To enhance the design pattern of the tattoo
- To make the tattoo last longer.

These tattoos stain the skin black and have the appearance of a real tattoo. Because black henna tattoo mixtures are often extemporaneously prepared by the artist with a variety of materials and sources, the actual concentrations of PPD and other ingredients may vary greatly.

Black henna can be distinguished from red henna in that:

- It is dark brown or black (pure red henna is green-grey in color)
- Does not change color when moistened (henna turns orange when moistened)
- Fixed on the skin in less than 1 hour (henna needs between 2 hr and 12 hr to be fixed on the skin.[21]

Most patients with an allergic reaction become sensitized to PPD in the tattoo itself. Incubation periods (the time between application of the tattoo and the first signs of dermatitis) were usually between 8 days and 14 days, but, in many instances of active sensitization, short incubation periods of 4–7 days have been observed, especially in children, this is attributed to the sensitizing properties of PPD.[22] The concentrations of PPD range from 4.28% to 27.24% in various preparations.

CONCLUSION

In summary, the majority of tattoo inks are a mixture of not only containing labeled colorants but also a large variety of known and unknown molecules. The tattoo artist makes their preferred blends by mixing different complex pigments and by adding thinners and additives. In such a situation it is difficult to find the cause of allergic reaction. To minimize the public health risks, one should expect strict regulation concerning materials used to implant into the human body and draw a parallel between tattoo inks and medicine. Besides the toxicological aspects, the sterility of the products is another point of concern. Many of the body art practitioners have only elementary knowledge about sterility, and tattoo can be a major source of infection.

REFERENCES

1. Von Christa de Cuyper, Maria Luisa Cotapos. Dermatologic Complications of Body Art, 1st edition. Berlin Heidelberg: Springer-Verlag; 2009.
2. Wenzel SM, Rittmann I, Landthaler M, et al. Adverse reactions after tattooing: review of the literature and comparison to results of a survey. Dermatology. 2013;226:138-47.
3. Lehmann G, Pierchalla P. Tattooing dyes. Derm Beruf Umwelt. 1988;36(5):152-6.
4. Ross EV, Yashar S, Michaud N, et al. Tattoo darkening and nonresponse after laser treatment: a possible role for titanium dioxide. Arch Dermatol. 2001;137(1):33-7.
5. Cui Y, Spann AP, Couch LH, et al. Photodecomposition of pigment yellow 74, a pigment used in tattoo inks. Photochem Photobiol. 2004;80(2):175-84.
6. Baeumler W, Vasold R, Lundsgaard J, et al. Chemicals used in tattooing and permanent make up products. In: Papameletiou D, Schwela D, Zenie A, Baeumler W (Eds). Workshop on the Technical/Scientific and Regulatory Issues on the Safety of Tattoos, Body Piercing and Related Practices. European Commission, Ispra. pp. 21-37.
7. Engel E, Vasold R, Santarellei F, et al. Tattooing of skin results in transportation and light Induced decomposition of tattoo pigments – a first quantification in vivo using a mouse model. Exp Dermatol. 2009;19(1):54-60.
8. Gopee NV, Roberts DW, Webb P, et al. Migration of intradermally injected quantum dots to sentinel organs in mice. Toxicol Sci. 2007;98(1):249-57.
9. North, Ministry of Health (2001) Tattoo and permanent make-up colorants. An exploratory examination of: chemical and microbiological composition, Legislation, Report no ND COS 012.
10. Timko AL, Miller CH, Johnson FB, et al. In vitro quantitative chemical analysis of tattoo pigments. Arch Dermatol. 2001;137(2):143-7.
11. Regensburger J, Lehner K, Maisch T, et al. Tattoo inks contain polycyclic aromatic hydrocarbons that additionally generate deleterious singlet oxygen. Exp Dermatol. 2010;19:e275-e281.
12. Krutak L. Spiritual skin: magical tattoos and scarification. Germany: Edition Reuss; 2013.
13. Cui Y, Spann AP, Couch LH, et al. Photodecomposition of pigment yellow 74, a pigment used in tattoo inks. Photochem Photobiol. 2004;80(2):175-84.
14. Vasold R, Engel E, Konig B, et al. Health risks of tattoo colors. Anal Bioanal Chem. 2008;391(1):9-13.
15. Kluger N, Phan A, Debarbieux S, et al. Skin cancers arising in tattoos: coincidental or not? Dermatology. 2008;217:219-22.

16. Pfirrmann G, Karsai S, Roos S, et al. Tattoo removal – state of the art. J Dtsch Dermatol Ges. 2007;5(10):889-97
17. Christa de Cuyper, Maria Luisa Cotapos. Dermatologic Complications with Body Art: Tattoos, Piercings and Permanent. pg 24. Springer, Newyork, 2010.
18. Kazandjieva J, Grozdev I, Tsankov N. Temporary henna tattoos. Clin Dermatol. 2007;25(4):383-7.
19. Basas CG. Henna tattooing: cultural tradition meets regulation. Food Drug Law J. 2007;62:779-803.
20. Raupp P, Hassan JA, Varughese M, et al. Henna causes life threatening haemolysis in glucose-6-phosphate dehydrogenase deficiency. Arch Dis Child. 2001;85:411-2.
21. Almeida PJ, Borrego L, Pulido-Melian E, et al. Quantification of p-phenylenediamine and 2-hydroxy-1,4-naphthoquinone in henna tattoos. Contact Dermatitis. 2011;66:33-7.
22. Kligman A. The identification of contact allergens by human assay. J Invest Dermatol. 1966;47:393-402.

Chapter 4

Psychosocial Aspects of Tattoos

Smitha Prabhu S

INTRODUCTION

Tattooing is an art known to humankind since prehistoric times when the Paleolithic man decorated himself with scars made of flint knife, and it serves many purposes like ornamentation of the body, assertion of ideas and beliefs, exhibiting affection for the loved one, showing allegiance to certain sects, and even to increase self-esteem. Occasionally tattoos also mask defects like a vitiligo patch or a bad scar, or even a mentally perceived inadequacy. In certain African cultures the number and intricacy of tattoos indicate gender, physical age, mental maturity and even stature of individual in the social strata.[1]

The psychology and sociology of tattooing has been well-studied and there are varied and conflicting opinions. Tattooing has been considered as a primitive substitute for clothing, as a desire to beautify the body, a way of exhibiting bravado and the urge to identify with the in-crowd.[2]

TYPES OF INDIVIDUALS WHO GET TATTOO

Before the 1960s, tattoos remained culture specific and ritualistic. American seamen were the first group of individuals to attain tattoos, closely followed by bikers. Later, fraternity boys and celebrities took up the trait, and by the 21st century tattooing has become a common mainstream decorative activity, so much so that it has been labeled "modern day social branding".

There is a high incidence of tattooing in delinquents, people with personality disorders and prisoners. Tattooing is a sign of elevated "status" and exhibition of masochistic personality. Prisoners with tattoo were shown to be more narcissistic, more positive about their body image and had less guilt associated with sex.[3] Mostly it is normal people who undergo tattooing as a whim or fancy. The Harris Poll survey on tattoos in America showed that around 21% of people had a tattoo, and most were in the age group of 30–39. About one-third of tattooed people felt tattoos made them strong, sexy and attractive.[4] Males undergo more tattooing and the ratio is 5:1. Tattooing is mostly undertaken during vacations and while intoxicated.[5]

A German study on personality differences showed that tattooed individuals are more extroverted, sensation seeking and are in the search of a unique identity.[6] Adults with tattoo are shown to be more sexually active, with likelihood of more high-risk behaviors in various studies.

PSYCHOLOGICAL IMPORTANCE TO THE INDIVIDUAL

The factors for getting body tattooed vary from individual to individual. A decision toward getting a tattoo involves these three elements in varying degrees: (1) symbolism of the act, (2) exhibitionistic and (3) masochistic attitudes.[5]

The main factors behind getting tattooed are:
- Rebellion and expression of individuality (Figs. 4.1 and 4.2)
- Enhancement of appearance and sexual attraction
- Love of art and creativity
- As a pictorial representation of some personal significance

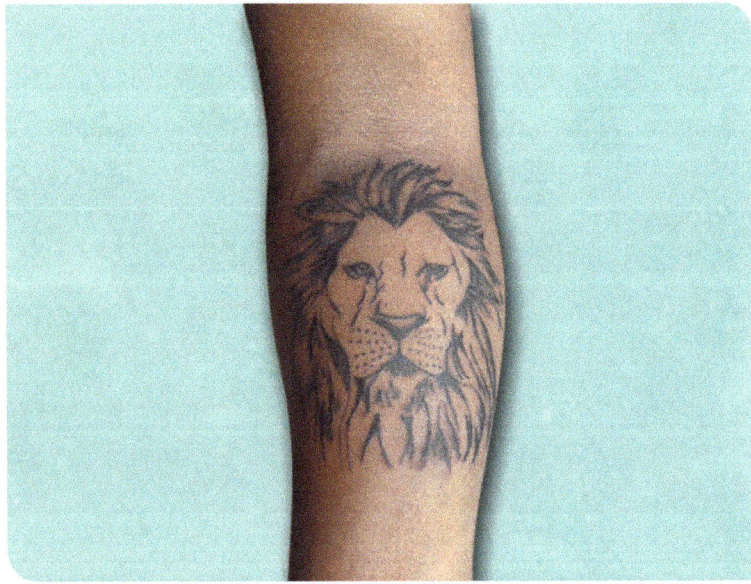

Fig. 4.1: Lion tattoo conveying courage, strength, pride and royalty.
Source: Dr Shashikumar BM.

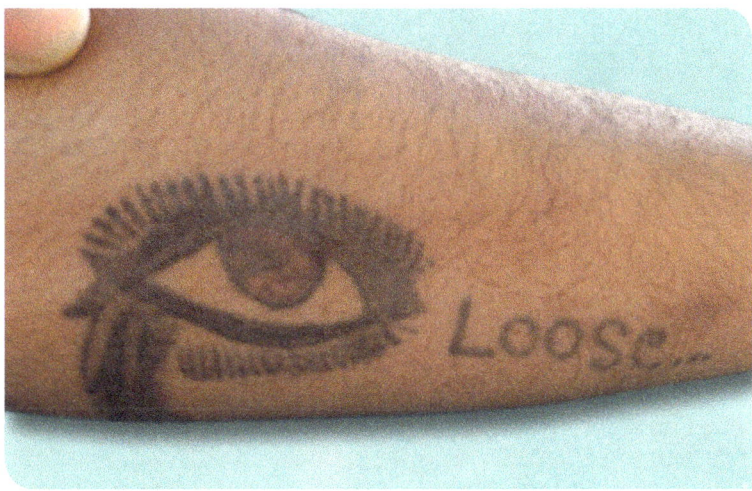

Fig. 4.2: Individual personality.
Source: Dr Shashikumar BM.

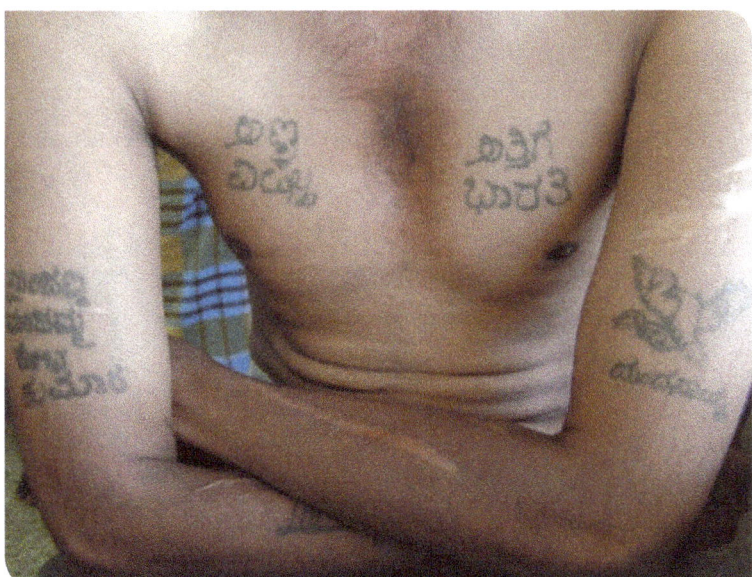

Fig. 4.3: Family members name tattoo.
Source: Dr Shashikumar BM.

- Remembering loved ones, family members (Fig. 4.3) or celebrity (Fig. 4.4)
- Group affiliation and commitment
- Cultural, spiritual or religious importance.

Some people also like to test their pain endurance or try to overcome the fear of needle by getting tattooed. Often it is done when in a state of

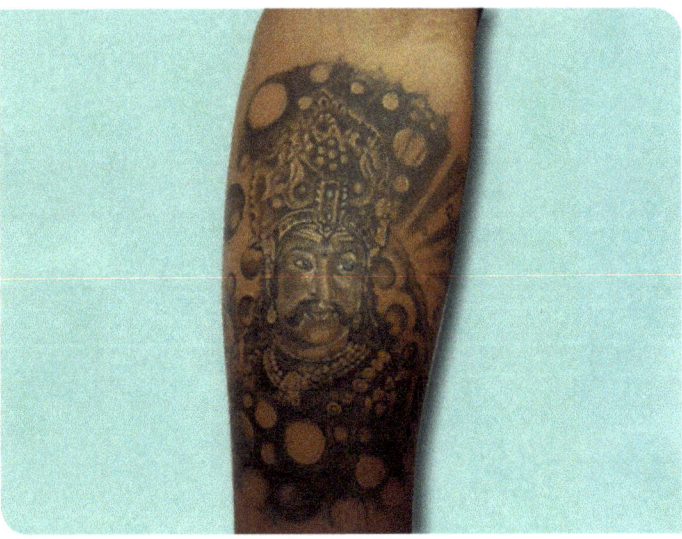

Fig. 4.4: Celebrity tattoo on the forearm.
Source: Dr Shashikumar BM.

intoxication or succumbing to peer pressure.[7] To most, tattoo signifies power and indestructibility. Immediately after tattooing, there is more body appreciation, higher self-esteem and lower anxiety. The tattooed person perceives himself as livelier and better than his peers and feels indestructible.

WHAT THE TATTOO SIGNIFIES ABOUT A PERSON?

Someone who gets a tattoo or personal, rather than religious or cultural purposes portrays themselves as a brave person who thinks of themselves as eternal, and is willing to change their body permanently. Tattooing increases the self-esteem in susceptible people. People who get tattoos done on prominent sites of their anatomy are attention seeking and want to stand out in a group.

Some groups and gangs have a mascot tattoo which enables individual members seem to belong closely to each other and to the group, and also enables members of large gangs to identify each other. Other reasons for getting a tattoo are memory of a loved one, displaying attitude or character trend like humor, love for literature, animal love, or to please a beloved of the opposite gender. The sexual character of tattooing is apparent in men who tattoo naked females on their forearms or trunk, and females in certain subcultures who tattoo their external genitalia to attract men.[2] A Bulgarian study considered unprofessional tattooing as symbols of autoaggression and self-infliction of injury, a means of resistance to authority and norms and a tendency to mimic the Western culture.[8]

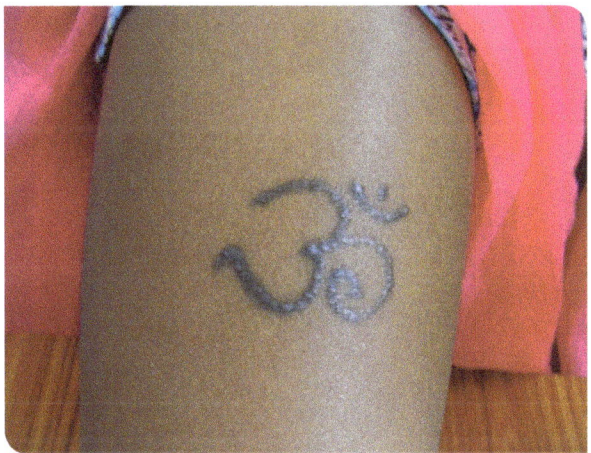

Fig. 4.5: Drawing of Om (Hindu religion tattoo).
Source: Dr Shashikumar BM.

Egoistic people draw attention to pertinent parts of their anatomy by tattooing beautiful images like butterflies and figurines. Tattoos depicting the Egyptian ankh, Hindu Om (Fig. 4.5), cross symbol and various deities in caricature soothe the psyche as well as impart a sense of indestructibility.[8] The decision to be pierced itself is an assertion of individuality and the design is often an escape from control and conformity. A person who submits to tattoo lives more in the present, and does not believe in the traditional earn and save concept of life.[9]

Psychologists consider tattooed individuals as narcissistic, uninhibited, impulsive, emotionally immature, neurotic people prone to exhibitionism and masochism and delinquency. Tattoos also compensate for physical and mental handicap.[10] There are also contradictory studies stating that tattoo seekers show integrated, adaptive and socially acceptable behavior patterns. People with multiple tattoos have more personality disorders including maladjustment, as compared to those with a single tattoo.[5]

In a certain subtype of individuals, who keep on acquiring tattoos and almost covering their whole bodies, it can be considered as an adaptive as well as addictive behavior (Figs. 4.6A to D).

COMMON TATTOO DESIGNS AND WHAT THEY SIGNIFY?

Tattoos have been broadly placed into three categories:[5]
1. Mnemonic tattoos.
2. Erotic or decorative tattoos.
3. Philosophical tattoos.

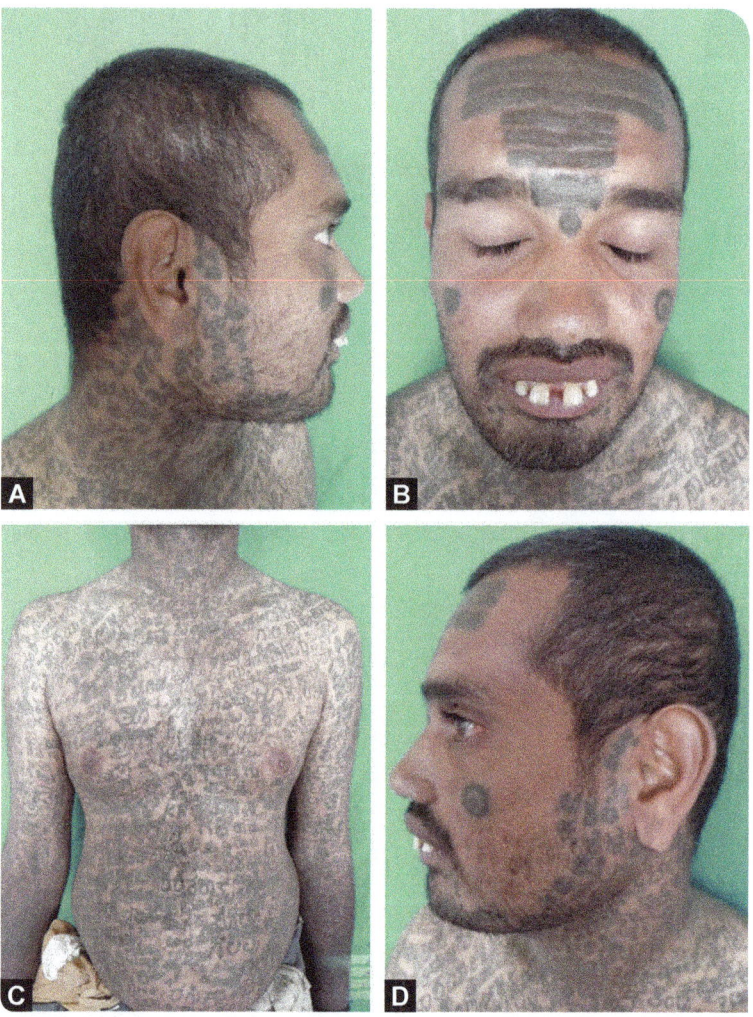

Figs. 4.6A to D: Whole body tattoo. He used to get tattooed in every fair he attends. *Source:* Dr Shashikumar BM.

Tattoos have been classified into various subclasses by Ferguson-Rayport et al. (Table 4.1):[11]

- A skull on the body suggests that one has conquered/is not afraid of death
- Teeth, fangs or jaws are used to intimidate others, especially by sports teams and gang members.

Tattooing is considered as a nonverbal means of communication. Offensive, abusive and erotic tattoos are often encountered in prisoners and army rejects who have neuropsychiatric problems.[5] There are studies correlating offensive tattoos to criminal behavior.

Table 4.1: Classification of tattoos.[11]

Type	Subtype	Example
1. Identification tattoos	• Emblems • Personal data • Life events	• Societies, committee, gangs • Initials, date of birth • Wedding, job
2. Love tattoos	• Idealized love • Mother • Sentimental • Pornographic	• Woman draped in flag, within a moon, etc. • Heart, flower, etc. inscribed with mother • Initials of lover • Nude woman, body parts
3. Bombastic and pseudoheroic tattoos		• Skull with cross bones • Dagger • Panther
4. Inviting fate		• Card with no. 13 • Horseshoe with good luck
5. Religious and commemorative		• Jesus • Cross • Hindu Om • Egyptian ankh
6. Private symbols		Significance is known only to the user
7. Miscellaneous		Animals, birds, flowers, butterflies

Tattoos indicating specific subtypes: the well-known Pachuco cross tattoo (a cross with three lines radiating upward, usually found on the web between the thumb and index finger) (Fig. 4.7) of Hispanic origin has been adopted by Western youth offenders.

"Jail house tattoos" are crude, often painfully etched into the skin and proclaim that one is brave and powerful, and is part of a larger group, rather than a lone individual. This is often seen in people belonging to prisons and camps. These often carry cryptic messages and identities.

In some female prisons, the passive lesbian partner is tattooed with the initials of her dominant lover on the right third finger. Worded tattoos often proclaim antisocial behavior (e.g. born to be a rebel, I hate police) and devout people have religious tattoos.

TATTOOS AND THE PSYCHE: INDIAN EXPERIENCE

There are no exhaustive studies or case reports on the psychology and sociology of tattooing in India. On personal interviews with patients with tattoos, varying responses given were:

• A book lover and music lover wanted to tattoo related themes on her inner wrist for her next birthday as she felt it will make her happy whenever she sees it.

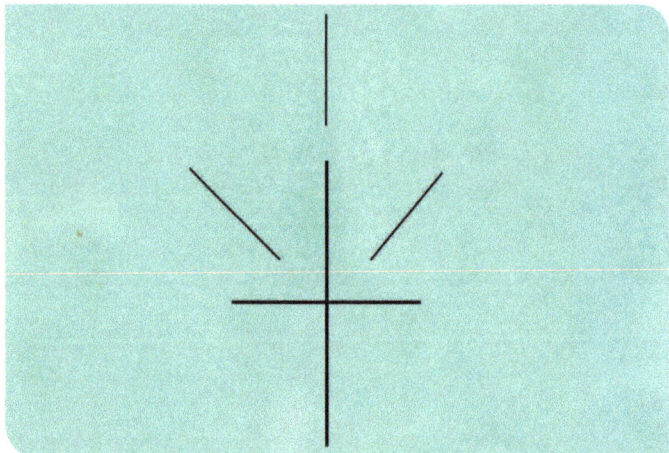

Fig. 4.7: The Pachuco Cross.

- One person said that his favorite rock star has a tattoo, and he too wanted it.
- A newly wedded couple got their partner's initials tattooed on their ring fingers in lieu of the traditional ring.
- A lady, who lost her mother, tattooed her mother's name surrounded by four stars, depicting herself and three siblings, on her wrist.
- A dog lover has tattooed paw prints on her arm to express eternal love for her dog.
- There were also multiple tattoos of Tibetan chakra, Hindu Om and Chinese alphabets which symbolized power and rebirth.
- One person with multiple tattoos said she is addicted to tattooing, and the pain of tattoo needle gives her a sense of serenity.
- A person has tattooed all his important dates in various parts of his body (birth, first day of job, marriage, separation).
- A girl tattooed a Phoenix after a bad romantic breakup.
- One man had name of his two daughters on each arm.

A highly intelligent writer, who on asking about his tattoo of his favorite character (Arya Stark of Game of Thrones fantasy book series), replied eloquently that "A tattoo is a kind of relationship, or so it felt. You realize that it is going to be there forever and taking a plunge to that kind of commitment means that the tattoo you want for yourself is something that defines way more than anything or anyone can make you feel and understand. May be its something that makes you feel adequate, something that makes you strong or sometimes its just there to complete nothing in particular. It makes you feel good, confident even and you are proud of whatever it is that is a part of your body now".

All these people had tattoos mainly on their wrists, arms and posterior neck.

TATTOO AND ENTERTAINMENT INDUSTRY

In 2008, "Ghajini", a hugely successful Indian film was released, which depicted an important role for tattoos: a man with anterograde amnesia who tattooed his body with different images whenever he gained fragments of memory, so as to recover his memory to avenge the death of his beloved. The Girl with the Dragon Tattoo is a psychological thriller novel by a Swedish author, which has a troubled criminal turned vigilante teenager, Lisbeth Salander, who has multiple piercings and tattoos, including a dragon tattoo prominently displayed on her left shoulder blade. She has had a troubled childhood and is socially aggressive.

TATTOO REMOVAL AND PSYCHOLOGICAL BEHAVIOR

Although the craze for tattooing is on the rise, an equal number of people desire tattoo removal and many a times they are in a hurry to do so for various personal, social or occupational reasons. Getting tattoos of the names of the current love interest leads to a lot of psychological distress if there is a change of heart. Dissatisfaction or boredom with an existing tattoo is the main reason sometimes for removal of tattoo. Feelings of low self-esteem, stigmatization and anxiety are common in patients seeking tattoo removal. Sometimes abnormal methods are employed in anger or frustration to get rid of tattoo or bad memory due to tattoo (Figs. 4.8 and 4.9). When not succeeded, frustration increases and goes to depression.

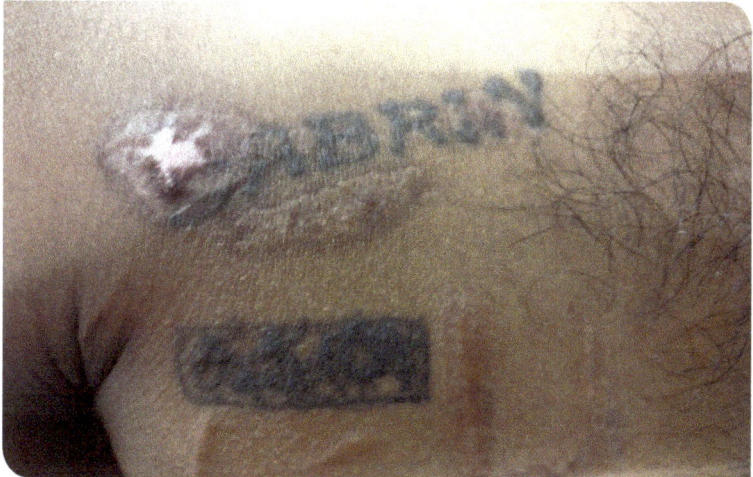

Fig. 4.8: Individual tried to erase the tattoo by burning the skin.
Source: Dr Shashikumar BM.

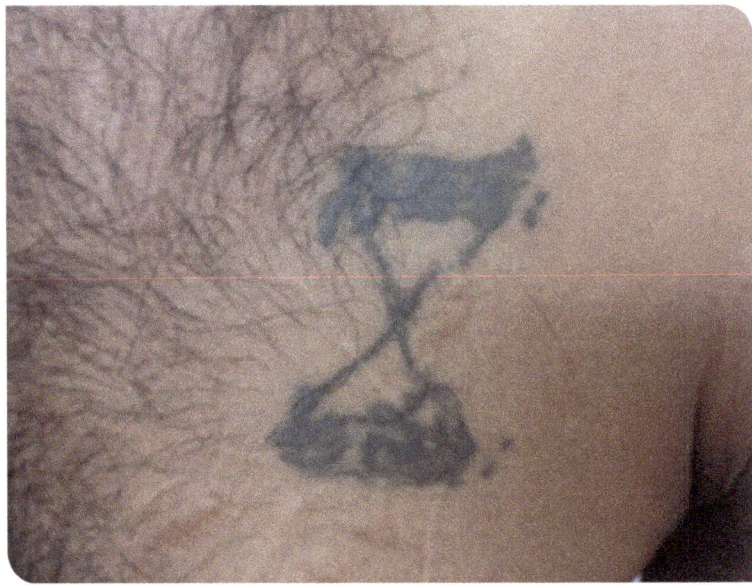

Fig. 4.9: Same patient when not succeeded retattooed the area to camouflage it. *Source:* Dr Shashikumar BM.

CONCLUSION

Tattooing is a growing form of body art, indulged in by people irrespective of gender, age or station in life. These serve varying purposes from mitigation of boredom, love for art, expression of ideals, love for living and nonliving objects, as well as belonging to a group or sect, and occasionally as a form of body harm or aggression. Tattoos are here to stay, and innovative means of expression are being explored day by day. Though majority of the persons indulging in tattooing are ordinary people from varying sects of life, an underlying psychological problem should be explored in those with multiple tattoos, large body area tattoos, images depicting violence and nudity and tattooing of unusual body parts.

REFERENCES

1. Nia S, Towers A. (2013). The psychological impact of tattoos. [online] Available from www.nwitimes.com/the-psychological-impact-of-tattoos/article_0c362 cc9-df4b-50a5-b937-a96c355966d4.html. [Accessed April, 2017].
2. Cohen MJ. Tattooing: some medical and psychological aspects. Br J Dermatol. 1927;39(7):290-7.
3. Mosher DL, Oliver WA, Dolgan J. Body image in tattooed prisoners. J Clin Psychol. 1967;23(1):31-2.

4. Burgemeester A. (2015). Psychology of tattoos, body piercings and sexual activity. [online] Available from psychologized.org/psychology-of-tattoos-body-piercings-and-sexual-activity/. [Accessed April, 2017].

5. Post RS. The relationship of tattoos to personality disorders. J Crim Law Criminol. 1968;59(4):516-24.

6. Swami V, Pietschnig J, Bertl B, et al. Personality differences between tattooed and non-tattooed individuals. Psychol Rep. 2012;111(1):97-106.

7. Bhat A. (2016). The psychology of body modification. [online] Available from www.speakingtree.in/blog/the-psychology-of-body-modification. [Accessed April, 2017].

8. Kazandjieva J, Kamarashev J, Kadurina M, et al. Unprofessional tattoos in Bulgaria—psychological aspects. J Eur Acad Dermatol Venereol. 1995;4(3):254-9.

9. Farrell K. (2013). If Tattoos Could Talk. Fangs, gangs, and the pangs of youth. [online] Available from www.psychologytoday.com/blog/swim-in-denial /201 310/if-tattoos-could-talk. [Accessed April, 2017].

10. Copes JH, Forsyth CJ. The tattoo: a social psychological explanation. Int Rev Mod Soc. 1993;23(2):83-9.

11. Ferguson-Rayport SM, Griffith RM, Straus EW. The psychiatric significance of tattoos. Psychiatr Q. 1955;29(1):112-31.

Chapter 5

Uses of Tattoos

Sukesh MS, Sujit Shanshanwal

INTRODUCTION

Tattooing involves the process of implantation of exogenous metabolically inert color fast pigments into the skin or mucous membranes. In this process, only pigment particles introduced through the skin surface, below the dermoepidermal junction, are retained by the dermal macrophages and fibroblasts where they reside permanently, producing an indelible change of the skin color under the form of a recognizable pattern or design.[1]

Historically, tattoos have been found on Egyptian mummies as an indication of worship to a God, and Roman gladiators are known to have used tattoos for identification.[2] Skin marking with pigments has been used by people for at least 4,000 years.[3] In the first half of the 20th century, tattooing was considered fashionable among royalty.[4] The first papers to document unequivocally medical application of tattooing in dermatology and ophthalmology appeared by the mid-1800s.[5-7] The word "tattoo" itself was introduced by Captain Cook (1796), who wrote of the Polynesian practice of inlaying black pigments under the skin, known popularly as *Tattow* in their native language.[8] During the past several decades, however, the public perception of tattooing has greatly evolved. Tattoos and other types of body art, such as piercing, have dramatically increased in popularity, especially among adolescents and young adults.[1]

TYPES OF TATTOOS

The American Academy of Dermatology distinguishes five types of tattoos: (1) traumatic tattoos, also called "natural tattoos" (that result from injuries, especially asphalt from road injuries or pencil lead); (2) amateur tattoos; (3) professional tattoos, both via traditional methods and modern tattoo machines; (4) cosmetic tattoos (also known as "permanent makeup"—mainly used for makeup and hiding or neutralizing skin discolorations, like enhancing eyebrows, lips, eyes, and even moles, usually with natural colors, as the designs are intended to resemble makeup; or placing artistic tattoos over the surgical scars); and (5) medical tattoos.[5]

USES OF TATTOO

The terms "micropigmentation" and "dermatography", which are both coined recently, convey the esthetic use of tattooing for medical purposes. It can ensure permanent camouflage in a wide range of dermatological diseases. It can also be a valuable finishing step in several surgical procedures in the fields of craniofacial surgery, plastic and reconstructive operations, cosmetic surgery procedures, and breast reconstruction.[1]

Tattooing has been used for medical alert purpose as a replacement for medical alert jewelry to alert first time responders regarding specific health conditions, blood group or DNR (do not resuscitate) directives. Training of emergency medical technicians includes recognition of such marks along with looking for medical alert necklaces and bracelets.[9,10]

Cosmetic Tattooing

It is the art of improving the appearance of eyelids, augmentation or replacement of eyebrows, and improvement of lip contour after trauma or surgery. Other potential fields of micropigmentation surgery include permanent eye lining, eyelash enhancement for sparse lashes, and nipple replacement by tattooing.[11]

Eyelid tattooing/blepharopigmentation is achieved by a single-pronged 23 or triple-pronged 27 needle coated with ferrous oxide pigment, moving rapidly in a reciprocating fashion. The pigment is implanted at the base of the eyelashes and between the lashes in dot like fashion, from lateral to medial canthus. The dots are applied sequentially, so that they barely overlap, which provides a subtle, fine line of pigmentation. It is recommended that both lower eyelids be tattooed first. In the upper eyelids a heavier line may be obtained by pigmenting two or more rows of dots that should be confluent, with the outer edges of each dot overlapping.[12] Complications related to this procedure are mostly reported in the ophthalmology literature, including long-lasting pigment spreading, eyelid margin necrosis, cilia loss, secondary cicatricial entropion and preseptal cellulitis.[13] Most commonly, these appear to be caused by improper technique. To avoid ocular injury, a protective shield is advised.[12,13]

The lip liner or full lip color can be done using micropigmentation to change the size and shape of the lips as well as to deepen their color.[14] It is a simpler and permanent technique than collagen implants for the creation of French lips. Many patients need permanent lip tattooing as a final step in lip rejuvenation surgeries, such as lip advancement and lip-lift, resurfacing, and autologous fat augmentation. Red dye is tattooed into the lip mucosa and over the vermillion border to advance the red color over the lips onto the glabrous skin.[15] Rare complications have been described with this procedure, such as contact dermatitis to pigment ingredients, contact granulomas, pseudoepitheliomatous hyperplasia, and a case of sarcoidosis.[16]

The eyebrows coloring aims to give the appearance of hair in the browline and more fullness for sparse eyebrows or creating an artificial brow when the hair is absent.[14] It can also be used for eyebrow reconstruction in conditions of resistant alopecia areata, trichotillomania, hypothyroidism, cicatricial alopecia, etc.

Although the technique of permanent makeup is fairly simple, it can give satisfactory results only in experienced hands and necessitates close observation and simple precautions. A previous history of Koebnerizing skin disorder, allergies to makeup products or to other substances, and skin infections (herpes simplex) should be carefully collected before planning the procedure.[17-24]

Dermatography/Application of Tattooing Techniques in Dermatology

The tattooing procedure in dermatography consists of implantation of different colors through several consecutive sessions until complete matching of the color of the surrounding skin is obtained. The color pigments used consist of a mixture of ferric oxides, carbon black, titanium dioxide, and tartrazine. A series of 64 standard colors varying in intensity between 10% and 100% serve as a reference for specific applications and may be mixed to obtain different subtle shades.[17]

For the last 15 years, dermatography has been applied with excellent results in a wide range of indications, including hyperpigmentation and depigmentation caused by congenital defects, skin diseases, trauma, and after surgical interventions in plastic and reconstructive surgery and craniomaxillofacial surgery (Table 5.1).[18]

A common indication is its use for vitiligo which is the most common depigmenting disease (Figs. 5.1A to C). Patients partially responding or not responding to standard medical treatments are prescribed cosmetic camouflage creams, which, however, have the disadvantage of rubbing-off on areas where there is friction and sweating and need to be applied daily. Permanent tattooing has been introduced in practice to restore a pigmented appearance of lesional skin in localized stable vitiligo.[19] It has been observed that when the dye is applied to achromic areas, the pigment appears darker

Table 5.1: Indications for dermatography as a primary and adjuvant treatment.[18]

Primary treatment

- Alopecia areata
- Areola- and mammillary reconstruction
- Depigmentation and hyperpigmentation
- Eyebrow reconstruction
- Endoscopic marking of colon tumors
- External marking of endoprostheses
- Hemangioma
- Hypertrophic and atrophic scars
- Keloid formation
- Klippel-Trenaunay-Weber syndrome
- Pseudo hair formation
- Scar corrections
- Tattoo removal with penta-monogalloyl-glucose
- Trichotillomania
- Verrucae vulgares
- Vitiligo
- Xanthelasmata

Adjuvant treatment

- Adamantinoma—cancrum oris
- Ameloblastoma
- Burns
- Cleft lip and palate
- Ectodermal dysplasia
- Marking for a Bridley bladder pacemaker
- Marking of resection areas
- Scleroderma
- Seathre-Chotzen syndrome
- Skin transplants
- Sturge-Weber syndrome
- Transplants in head and neck
- Tumor marking in the mucosa

compared to the adjoining skin on initial application but there is dramatic esthetic improvement with only moderate degree of fading at 6 weeks.[2] The results from several reported studies showed excellent color matching in cutaneous[20] mucosal[21] and mucocutaneous vitiligo.[20,22]

Tattooing can also be used in genetic leukoderma like piebaldism and halo nevus (tattooing of the depigmented zone followed by electrocauterization of the nevus part),[23] post-traumatic depigmented scars or chemical leukoderma.

It has also been used to successfully camouflage port wine stains and capillary hemangiomas. Convay et al. have reported satisfaction in 84% patients from a total of 996 cases.[24]

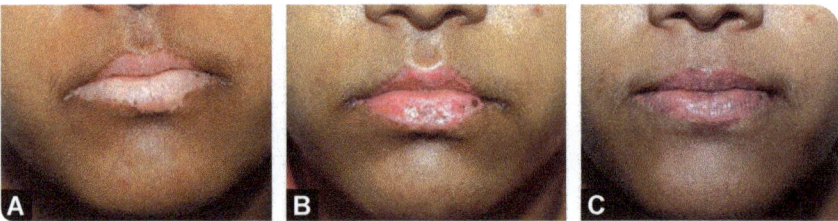

Figs. 5.1A to C: Micropigmentation for lip vitiligo (A) Preprocedure; (B) after 1st session; and (C) after 2nd showing uniform matching color of lip.
Source: Dr Madhura C, Consultant dermatologist, Cutis Academy of Cutaneous Sciences.

Scalp micropigmentation (SMP) is a recent addition to the usage of tattoo to create the illusion of hair over scalp in hair loss conditions (described in detail below).

Syringomas, benign appendageal tumors of the intraepidermal eccrine sweat duct, have been successfully treated by means of tattooing followed by Q-switched Alexandrite laser.[25] The surface of the syringoma lesions was first de-epithelialized by vaporization with a clear pulse carbon dioxide laser, after which, iontophoresis with black ink was applied, followed by two-three shots of Q-switched Alexandrite laser on the tattooed papules. With this method, the black ink was used as photosensitizer for targeting the ductal adenomas that allowed the damage to the neighboring normal tissue to be avoided.

Tattooing may be a valuable finishing step in several surgical procedures in the fields of craniofacial surgery, plastic and reconstructive operations, cosmetic surgery procedures, and in breast reconstruction.[18] Dermatography has been successfully applied for correcting the color mismatch and reducing the scars in patients operated for unilateral and bilateral cleft lip and palate. In cases who need to undergo mastectomy, tattooing has been used for construction of the nipple areola complex as a final step of the breast reconstruction process. Postprocedure patients need to be informed the pigment might fade over time and they might require re-tattooing.[10]

Tattooing has also been used for several other medical indications like tattooing for corneal scarring, marking the target area prior to radiation therapy, endoscopic tattooing prior to gastrointestinal surgeries to guide the surgeon in locating the affected area.[10]

Tattooing Procedure in General

- Appropriate selection of patient explaining the procedure.
- Obtaining informed consent and preprocedure photographs.
- Avoid taking aspirin, nonsteroidal anti-inflammatory drugs (NSAIDs) such as motrin, vitamin E, ginger, ginkgo biloba and ginseng 10–14 days

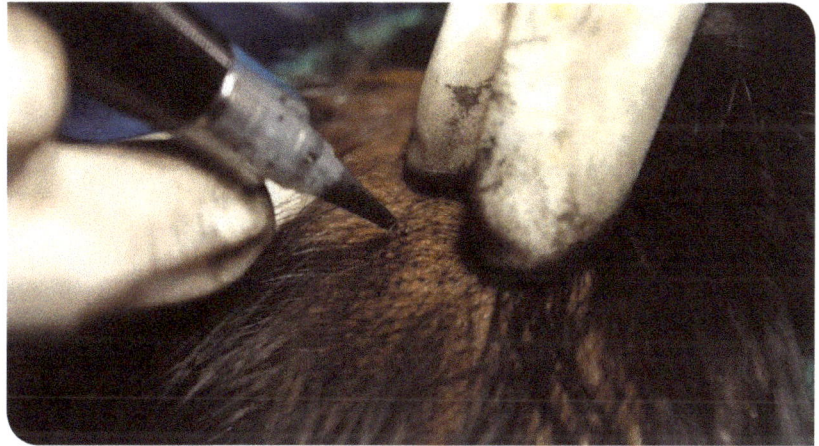

Fig. 5.2: Micropigmentation of scalp showing holding of tattoo gun.
Source: Dr Madhura C, Consultant dermatologist, Cutis Academy of Cutaneous Sciences.

prior to the procedure. These drugs and herbs may cause excessive bleeding or bruising.
- Local anesthesia is usually not required. However, in uncooperative or apprehensive patients topical anesthesia may be used.
- Clean and prepare the treated area.
- Set up the machine by selecting appropriate needle number, needle length, and rotor speed.
- The pigment is taken in sterile plastic well and the conical tip of the activated handle is dipped into the ink whereby the ink is sucked into the chamber around the needle by capillary action.
- The handle of the tattoo machine is held vertically in a pen-holding fashion perpendicular to the surface of the skin and the pigmented is placed as needed (Fig. 5.2).
- At regular intervals, the tip has to be dipped in the ink to refill the chamber as needed.

Scalp Micropigmentation

Hair loss is one of the most common problems encountered by dermatologists in clinical practice. The main concern for the patient is the visibility of the scalp skin which occurs due to the loss of density and thickness thereby making the contrast between the skin and hair more prominent. Medical or surgical line of therapy may not always be sufficient to provide the density to the patient. In such cases, tattooing can be used as a concealer to decrease this contrast between hair and skin. SMP is an advanced form of tattooing by placing numerous microdots and thereby creating an illusion of hair.

In 2001, Traquina et al. were the first to report use of micropigmentation on scalp in 62 patients with scalp scars.[26] However, the method used was crude and the pigmentation was quite detectable. Over time, there has been considerable refinement in the process of SMP.

The outcome of SMP depends on several variables like the quality of the target skin, the parameters used on the machine, dye used and the method with which the procedure is performed. SMP is performed by using single or triple pronged needles depending on the desired size dots. Also, it is important to note that the density of dots does not need to match the number of follicular openings as the pigments tend to diffuse in the skin after placement. These dots should be placed in a randomly, instead of a regular and linear grid fashion, in order to avoid the visibility of a distinct pattern and thereby avoiding the pattern from being caught by the naked eye easily.

The needle should be introduced into the skin at a perpendicular angle to ensure formation of regular sized round microdots. The needle should be introduced slightly beyond the dermoepidermal junction to ensure the deposition of pigment in the upper part of the dermis. If the pigment is deposited deep there is greater diffusion which results in a patchy appearance. On the other hand, if the pigment is deposited too superficially in the epidermis it shall be washed off with the epidermal turnover. The authors prefer setting the speed of the rotor at 5,500–6,500 cycles per minute and limiting the contact time of needle with the skin to 0.5–1.0 seconds. The pigment that is deposited is taken by the dermal macrophages and fibroblasts where they tend to continue residing in a predominantly per vascular location.[27]

In cases of atrophic or scarred skin, it is preferable to first perform a test patch to ensure adequate placement of pigment. It may be needed to increase the contact time of the needle with increased penetration into the skin due to the fibrosis and lack of blood supply in the target area.

The operator needs to be aware that the final pigment appearance will be less than the immediate postoperative condition as the pigment that is deposited in the epidermal tract will be washed off over the initial couple of weeks. Also, when selecting the patient, it is important to counsel regarding the need for touch up sessions that would be needed as the pigment tends to fade over time.

Scalp micropigmentation can serve as an excellent therapeutic option in various types of alopecias. It can be used in androgenetic alopecia in both men (Figs. 5.3A and B) and women as well as in patients who have undergone hair transplant further augment the results by providing a camouflage. It can be used for the post-hair transplant scars of both follicular unit extraction and follicular unit transplantation. SMP can be used in cicatricial

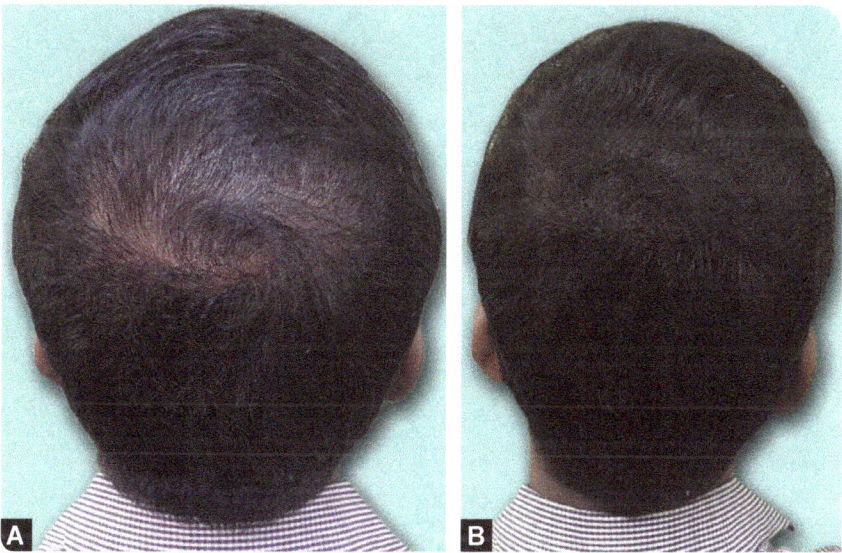

Figs. 5.3A and B: Pre- and postimages of micropigmentation done for male pattern baldness with vertex thinning.
Source: Dr Rachita Dhurat, Prof. & Head, Dept. of Dermatology, LTM Medical College, Mumbai.

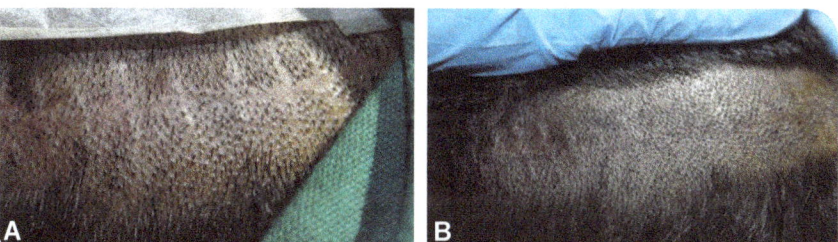

Figs. 5.4A and B: Figures showing micropigmentation of scar in scalp (A) Preprocedure scar; and (B) complete micropigmentation of scar.
Source: Dr Madhura C, Consultant dermatologist, Cutis Academy of Cutaneous Sciences.

alopecias (Figs. 5.3 to 5.5) which could be congenital, post-traumatic or secondary to pathologic process.[28]

Scalp micropigmentation should be avoided in patients who have skin diseases which may be exaggerated due to Koebnerization, have a history of reaction to black ink, inherited or acquired blood disorders, history or atypical mole, personal or family history of melanoma, and immunosuppressive conditions or intake of immunosuppressive medications.

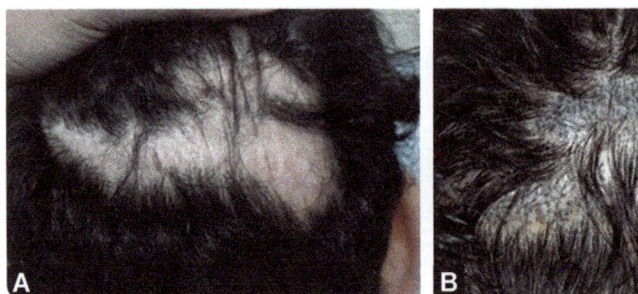
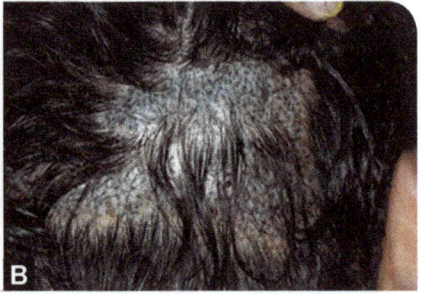

Figs. 5.5A and B: Pre- and postimages of micropigmentation done for cicatricial alopecia.
Source: Dr Madhura C, Consultant dermatologist, Cutis Academy of Cutaneous Sciences.

Complications of Medical Tattooing

In comparison to the widespread practice of tattooing done in the western countries, the incidence of side effects is negligible. Complications that occur are mostly when the procedure is not performed under aseptic precautions. Complications seen are infections (bacterial, mycobacterial, fungal or viral), koebnerization, granuloma reactions, benign lesions like epidermal cysts or milia and in rare cases malignant lesions like malignant melanoma, and basal cell or squamous cell carcinoma.[29] In pregnant or breast feeding women, the risk to complications is same as any other individual. However, for the fetus, the risk of transmission of infection or effect of toxicity due to the chemicals across the placenta or breast milk has not been evaluated and, hence, the procedure is best avoided in such cases.[28] The few case reports indicating a very rare occurrence of malignant lesions that have been mentioned could most possibly be coincidental without actual association with the procedure.[29]

CONCLUSION

Tattooing procedure is a valuable addition to the armamentarium of therapeutic options which can be used for many indications in dermatology. The utility of scalp micropigmentation procedure is on a rise. Tattooing procedure is relatively easy, provides good camouflage, and is generally devoid of any significant adverse effects, in experienced hands. The proper selection of cases is mandatory, and the dermatologists should be aware of the potential complications.

REFERENCES

1. Vassileva S, Hristakieva E. Medical applications of tattooing. Clin Dermatol. 2007;25(4):367-74.
2. Garg G, Thami GP. Micropigmentation: tattooing for medical purposes. Dermatol Surg. 2005;31(8 Pt 1):928-31.
3. Grumet GW. Psychodynamic implications of tattoos. Am J Orthopsychiatry. 1983;53:482-92.
4. Van der Velden EM, de Jong BD, van der Walle HB, et al. Tattooing and its medical aspects. Int J Dermatol. 1993;32:381-4.
5. Pauli: Ueber das Feuermaal und die einzigsichere Methode, disease ensteullungzuheilen. J Geburttsh. 1835;15:66-72.
6. Turell R, Marino AW. Technic of tattooing with mercury sulfide for pruritus ani. Ann Surg. 1942;115:126-30.
7. VonWecker L. Das Tätowiren der Hornhaut. Arch Augenheilkunde. 1872;2:84-7.
8. Earley MJ. Basal cell carcinoma arising in tattoos: a clinical report of two cases. Br J Plast Surg. 1983;36:258-9.
9. "Tattoos, Body Piercings, and Other Skin Adornments". Aad.org. Retrieved 5 April 2012.
10. Glassy CM, Glassy MS, Aldasouqi S. Tattooing: medical uses and problems. Cleveland Clin J Med. 2012;79(11):761-70.
11. Ortonne JP, Bose SK. Pigmentation: dyschromia. In: Baran R, Maibach HI (Eds). Textbook of Cosmetic Dermatology, 3rd edition. London and New York: Taylor & Francis; 2005. pp. 406-7.
12. Patipa M. Eyelid tattooing. Dermatol Clin. 1987;5:335-48.
13. Konuk O, Evereklioglu C, Handur A, et al. Protective eye shield can prevent corneal trauma during micropigmentation for permanent cosmetic eyeliner. J Eur Acad Dermatol Venereol. 2004;18:642-3.
14. Oumeish YO. The cultural and philosophical concepts of cosmetics in beauty and art through the medical history of mankind. Clin Dermatol. 2001;19:375-86.
15. Fulton Jr JE, Rahimi DA, Helton P, et al. Lip rejuvenation. Dermatol Surg. 2000;26:470-5.
16. Yesudian PD, Azurdia RM. Scar sarcoidosis following tattooing of the lips treated with mepacrine. Clin Exp Dermatol. 2004;29:552-3.
17. Van der Velden EM, De Jong BD, Van der Walle HG, et al. Cosmetic tattooing as a treatment of port-wine stains. Int J Dermatol. 1993;32:372-5.
18. Van der Velden EM, Defranco J, Ijsselmuiden OE, et al. Dermatography: a review of 15 years of clinical applications in surgery. Int J Cosmet Surg Aesthet Dermatol. 2001;3:151-9.
19. Mutalik S, Ginzburg A. Surgical management of stable vitiligo: a review with personal experience. Dermatol Surg. 2000;26:248-54.
20. Halder RM, Pham HN, Breadon JY, et al. Micropigmentation for the treatment of vitiligo. J Dermatol Surg Oncol. 1989;15:1092-8.
21. Center JM, Mancini S, Baker GI, et al. Management of gingival vitiligo with the use of a tattoo technique. J Periodontol. 1998;69:724-8.
22. Singal A, Thami GP, Bhalla M. Watchamaker's pin-vise for manual tattooing of vitiligo. Dermatol Surg. 2004;30:203-4.
23. Mahajan BB, Geeta G. Tattooing with electrocauterization: a cosmetically acceptable therapeutic modality for a single halo nevus. Indian J Dermatol Venereol Leprol. 2002;68:288-9.

24. Conway H, McKinney P, Climo M. Permanent camouflage of vascular nevi of the face by intradermal injection of insoluble pigments (tattooing): experience through twenty years with 1022 cases. Plast Reconstr Surg. 1967;40:457-62.

25. Park HJ, Lim SH, Kang HA, et al. Temporary tattooing followed by Q-switched alexandrite laser for the treatment of syringomas. Dermatol Surg. 2001;27:28-30.

26. Traquina AC. Micropigmentation as an adjuvant in cosmetic surgery of the scalp. Dermatol Surg. 2001;27:123-8.

27. Rassman WR, Pak JP, Kim J, et al. Scalp micropigmentation: a concealer for hair and scalp deformities. J Clin Aesthet Dermatol. 2015;8(3):35-42.

28. Park JH, Moh JS, Lee SY, et al. Micropigmentation: camouflaging scalp alopecia and scars in Korean patients. Aesthetic Plast Surg. 2014;38(1):199-204.

29. Kaatz M, Elsner P, Bauer A. Body-modifying concepts and dermatologic problems: Tattooing and piercing. Clin Dermatol. 2008;26:35-44.

Chapter 6

Complications of Tattoos and its Management

Shashikumar BM

> *"The main complication of tattooing is regret"*
> —Nicolas Kluger

INTRODUCTION

Tattooing is an ancient practice and was popular among tribes. It has gained popularity and became a fashion statement in today's world. Also, there is a growing interest about tattoos among newer generation. India has witnessed phenomenal western trend among youths, which has contributed to this growing trend, consequently to increased reports of adverse reactions.

Broadly, tattoo can be classified as temporary, which lasts for weeks or permanent which lasts for life. Permanent tattooing can be of three types— (1) medical, (2) cosmetic (decorative tattoos and permanent makeup) or (3) traumatic tattoos.[1] All types of tattooing are associated with complications, but incidence is more with decorative tattoo done with unprofessional hands.

PREVALENCE

The prevalence of tattooing among general population varies with age, country and religion but the exact prevalence is unknown. The USA national prevalence rate of tattooing is 24% in the age group of 18–50 years.[2] A 2012 Harris interactive online poll indicated that 14% of the USA adults had one or more tattoos in 2008, and this proportion increased to 21% in 2012.[3] In Europe, the prevalence of tattoo among general population is about 12% but high prevalence was noted in Luxembourg (60%), Hungary (50%) and Cyprus (30%).[4] The exact prevalence in India is not known, but the same trend is continuing in India in recent days with increased number of people accepting tattooing.

Many reports of adverse reactions to tattoo are pouring nowadays but they are mainly case series and isolated case reports. Exact incidence of adverse reactions to tattoo is lacking as less number of patients approach dermatologists for the treatment, as many are trivial. Also, steroid creams are prescribed by tattoo artists to ameliorate acute transient reaction, which is often more common or as a routine practice.

A survey from Germany revealed an overall cutaneous adverse events and systemic reactions of 67.5% and 6.6%, respectively.[5] Another study from Germany by Kazandjieva et al. estimated the prevalence of complications in their series of 234 tattooed patients as 2.1%.[6]

TYPES OF TATTOO REACTIONS

Complications to tattoo may occur due to pigment or due to procedure. It may arise both with medical and decorative tattooing, but it is more with later. Both permanent and temporary tattoo may cause complication.

Complications of the permanent tattooing may be classified as:
- Cutaneous complications
- Extracutaneous complications.

Cutaneous Complications

Cutaneous complications related to tattoos are most common compared to systemic involvement. There is no concrete ways of classification of cutaneous adverse reactions after tattooing due to overlap between reactions, delay at appearance and presentations. Table 6.1 describes many ways of classification, but etiopathological classification is more useful.

Transient reactions, during the procedure and while healing, are the most common reactions and need no attention. Immediate postprocedure, client may experience acute aseptic inflammatory reaction of variable intensity, in the form of pain, tenderness, erythema, induration and edema (Fig. 6.1) ("peau d'orange" appearance with dilatation of the hair follicles of the tattooed skin). The tattoo heals within 2–3 weeks with superficial crusts, and the ink retained in the epidermis is shed as the epidermis peels away (Figs. 6.2A and B).[7,8]

Other abnormal reactions during acute phase along with its management are enumerated in Table 6.2.

Cutaneous Infections

Skin infections associated with tattoos are more frequently recognized as public health concern. These may range from simple folliculitis to septic shock and death (Table 6.3).[9] Infectious complications accounts for 0.5–6%

Duration of disease	Time of onset	Etiopathological
Acute (<3 months) Chronic (>3 months)	Early—infections Late—malignancy, hypersensitivity reactions	• Transient acute inflammatory reaction • Infection • Allergic • Malignancy • Skin disease localized in tattooed area • Interference with medical devices and imaging • Psychosocial complications • Complications of tattoo removal • Miscellaneous

Table 6.1: Types of classification of tattoo complications.

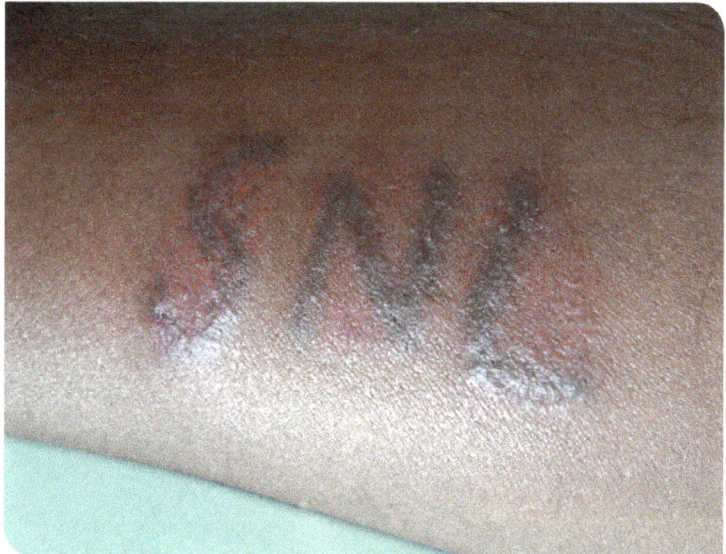

Fig. 6.1: Erythema and edema immediately after tattooing.

among tattooed people.[5,10-12] Many of the infectious complications seen secondary to tattoo are because of:
• Use of contaminated tattoo ink
• Inadequate disinfection of the skin
• Scratching during healing leading to superinfection.

Trauma to the skin secondary to tattooing will help to bypass the cutaneous barrier leading to local skin infections. In most cases, such mild-to-moderate superficial skin infections remain unreported since they are self-limiting or easily treated with proper aftercare, local disinfection measures and/or antibiotic therapy. Rarely, organism may enter main bloodstream causing systemic infections. The severity of infection depends on the virulence of the pathogen, the immune status of the person being tattooed and underlying diseases.[13]

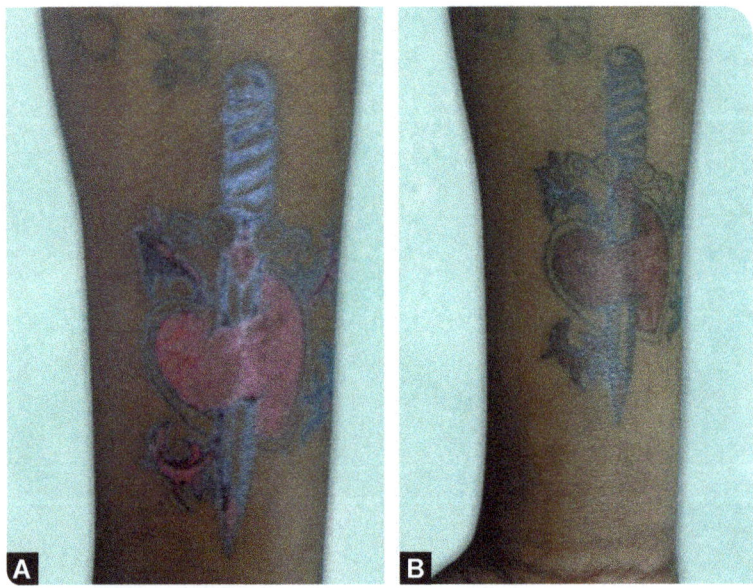

Figs. 6.2A and B: Immediate response on tattooing. (A) Day 1 after tattooing: Acute inflammatory changes - erythema and purpura seen; (B) Day 10 after tattooing. Inflammation subsides and superficial skin along with excess ink peels off.

Table 6.2: Immediate complication and its management.	
Complication	*Treatment and prevention*
Purpura	Self-resolving, rest
Hematoma	Rest, draining
Edema of foot, if done on large area of leg	Rest and foot-end elevation
Acute transient lymphadenopathy	Analgesics
Blue-foot or "tattoo blow-out"—"blurry halo" surrounding the main tattoo, due to spreading of tattoo pigment in the superficial subcutaneous plane	Laser tattoo removal
Acute contact dermatitis to topical anesthetic or antibiotic	Topical steroid
Secondary infection	Aseptic measures, oral and topical antibiotics
Delayed healing	

Table 6.3: Cutaneous infections.

Bacterial infections	
• Pyogenic infections	Folliculitis, furunculosis, erysipelas, necrotizing fasciitis, gangrene
• Nonpyogenic infections	Atypical mycobacteria, inoculation leprosy, inoculation tuberculosis, inoculation syphilis, tetanus
Viral infections	Viral wart (verruca vulgaris), molluscum contagiosum, herpes (herpes compunctorum)
Fungal	Tinea, sporotrichosis, zygomycosis, blastomycosis, mycetoma, *Aspergillus fumigatus*
Parasitic	Leishmaniasis

BACTERIAL INFECTIONS

Infection secondary to bacteria form the bulk of the infectious complications. It may be due to pyogenic infections, which are seen immediately within days or weeks or nonpyogenic infections, which manifests late.

Pyogenic infections: These are common and include superficial infections such as impetigo and folliculitis (Figs. 6.3 and 6.4) or deep bacterial skin infections presenting as erysipelas or cellulitis and systemic infections which may lead, in very rare cases, to life-threatening complications due to endocarditis, septic shock and multiorgan failure.[14] Acute pyogenic skin infections or bacteremia usually occur within a few days after placement of the tattoo and predominantly involve methicillin-resistant *Staphylococcus aureus* (MRSA) or methicillin-sensitive *Staphylococcus aureus* (MSSA), *Streptococcus* spp. and *Pseudomonas aeruginosa*. Many published bacteriological surveys have demonstrated presence of clinically relevant levels of bacteria in both opened and unopened tattoo ink bottles indicating contamination at the site of manufacturing. A systematic review by Dieckmann et al.[13] identified 2 of 39 colorants were contaminated with aerobic mesophilic bacteria. This is in addition to contamination at the tattoo parlor, which accounts for the large number of bacterial skin infections, following tattooing. In the past tattooist's, mainly amateur artists have used substances such as saliva, urine, dirty water, and tobacco juice topically during and after the tattooing process.[15]

Nonpyogenic infections: Onset of clinical signs of these infections is late, but chronic and persistent. It includes mycobacterial infections, syphilis, and tetanus.

- *Mycobacterial infections*: Cutaneous tuberculosis is rare nowadays. It can manifest as tuberculosis, leprosy, and atypical mycobacterias.
  - *Atypical mycobacterial infections*: Atypical mycobacterial infections, mainly rapidly growing mycobacteria infection, have emerged in

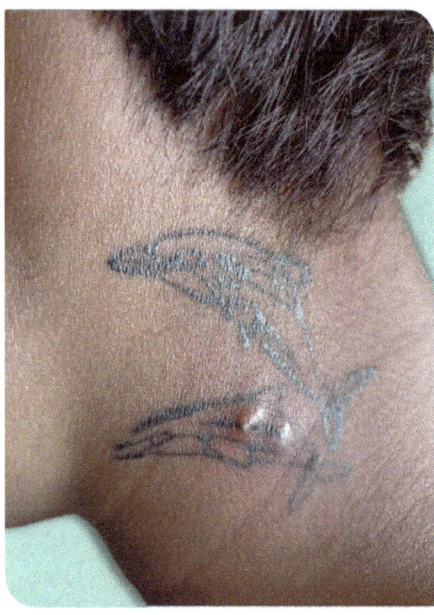

Fig. 6.3: Folliculitis followed after a week of tattooing.

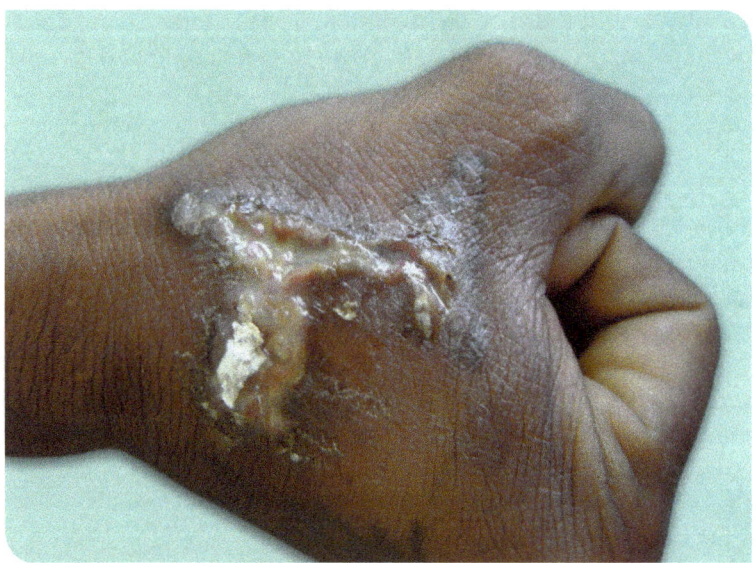

Fig. 6.4: Secondary infection with methicillin-resistant *Staphylococcus aureus*.

recent years. Several outbreaks in tattoo parlors have been reported in Scotland, France, the USA and Australia. A systemic review was carried out by Conaglen et al. in 2010, 25 reports from 11 countries were analyzed and identified 71 confirmed and 71 probable cases of rapidly growing mycobacteria infection. Of the confirmed case, 68% infections were due to *Mycobacterium chelonae, Mycobacterium haemophilum* (17%), *Mycobacterium abscessus* (8.4%), *M. chelonae abscessus, Mycobacterium immunogenum, Mycobacterium fortuitum* and unspecified mycobacteria were the other isolates.[16] The most postulated mechanisms were the use of nonsterile tap water to either dilute black ink to a gray "wash" or to clean tattooing equipment or due to environmental contamination of the tattoo ink.

Clinical presentation is varied and may present as chronic papules, pustules, lichenoid plaques, plaques with scales, which usually occur within 1–3 weeks after the procedure. Skin biopsies and bacterial cultures of skin and inks should be done and also identification to the species antimicrobial susceptibility. Appropriate antibiotics with or without concomitant surgical debridement for 3–6 months may be optimum. Intravenous imipenem or cefoxitin combined with amikacin as initial therapy accompanied by a macrolide antibiotic is the first choice.

- *Cutaneous tuberculosis*: It usually occurs following infection with *Mycobacterium tuberculosis* from an exogenous source or by endogenous spread from another site. Cutaneous tuberculosis in a tattoo has been reported after a tattooist with advanced pulmonary tuberculosis, mixed his saliva with the ink in the tattoo process.[17] Inoculation tuberculosis in the form of lupus vulgaris (Figs. 6.5 and 6.6) at tattooed area were reported in several Indian reports.[18,19] Biopsy, culture, Mantoux test, and polymerase chain reaction (PCR) are useful for making diagnosis. Treatment is as per Revised National Tuberculosis Control Program (RNTCP) category I comprising of Isoniazid (300 mg), Rifampicin (450 mg), Pyrazinamide (1,500 mg), Ethambutol (1,200 mg) for 2 months followed by Isoniazid (300 mg) and Rifampicin (450 mg) for 4 months (patients who weigh 60 kg or more receive additional Rifampicin 150 mg).

- *Leprosy*: Inoculation leprosy is mainly restricted to India. Lowe et al. first described the case of tattoo inoculated leprosy.[20] Ghorpade et al. reported 31 female cases of tattoo-inoculated leprosy in Chhattisgarh. Out of 31 cases, 29 were paucibacillary cases and two were multibacillary leprosy. In all of them, the first lesion of leprosy started over a tattoo mark. 25 cases had only single lesion of leprosy exclusively confined to tattoo marks. The duration between tattooing and appearance of first lesion in most of the cases varied from 10 years to 20 years.[21] He also reported tattoo inoculated borderline tuberculoid (BT) leprosy in upgrading reaction with prominent tattoo edema developing after starting paucibacillary multidrug therapy (PB MDT).[22]

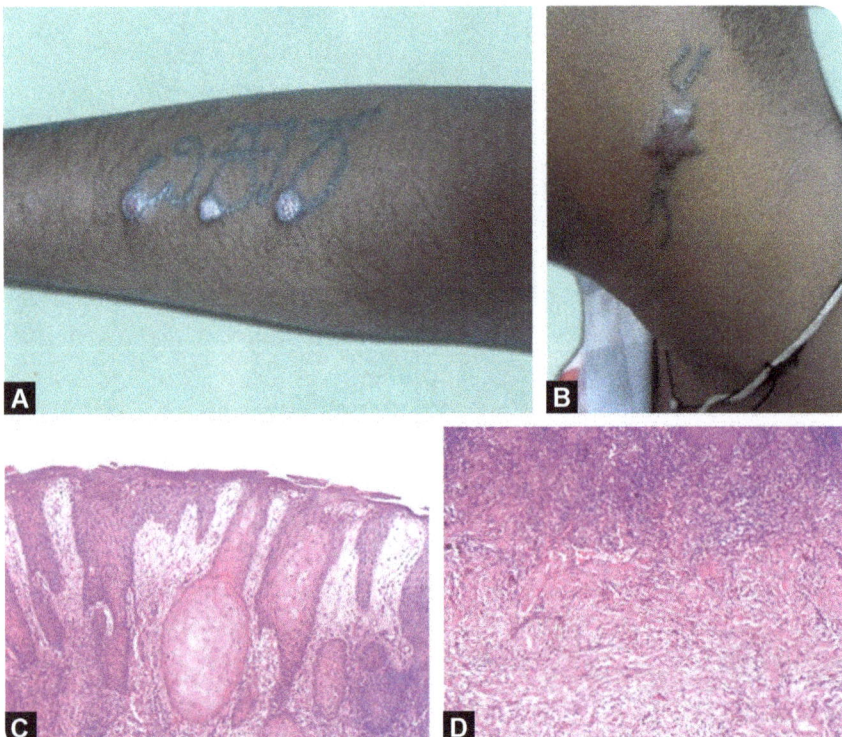

Figs. 6.5A to D: A case of lupus vulgaris over forearm and neck presented 2 months after tattooing. (A) Amateur tattoo was present since 5 years, added red color on the inferior margin 2 months back; (B) Red tattoo over the neck presenting as lupus vulgaris; (C) 100x, H and E, Patchy nodular tuberculoid granuloma; (D) 400×, H and E, granuloma shows lymphocytes, plasma cells, histiocytes, and epithelioid cells with occasional Langhans giant cells.

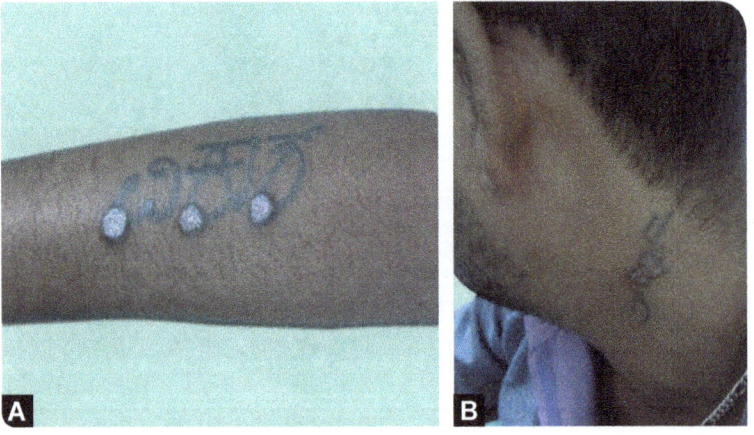

Figs. 6.6A and B: Resolution of tattoo induced lupus vulgaris after 6 months of antitubercular therapy.

- *Syphilis*: Syphilitic lesions have been described secondary to licking the tattoo needle by tattooist with oral primary or secondary syphilitic lesion, to suck out the residue of the pigment or to rewet the needle before dipping it into the dried pigment prior to skin puncturing.[23] Yuan described secondary syphilis on a red tattoo.[24] Benzathine penicillin is the drug of choice.

    Other bacterial infections: Other infections like chancroid, tetanus, and bacterial endocarditis have been reported following tattooing.[15,23]

Viral Infections

Warts:[7,15,25] Warts over the tattoo may manifest as verruca vulgaris (Fig. 6.7), verruca plana, or as warty growths. Lesions may occur from 1 month to 10 years after tattooing. Lesions may be variable in numbers and size, and may be restricted to one color. Besides contaminated instruments, modification of local immunity related to the ink itself, Koebner phenomenon during the procedure secondary to pre-existing clinical skin lesions may contribute.

Molluscum contagiosum: It is also a common viral infection associated with tattooing. Many case reports have followed the first case report by Foulds.[26] Treatment options include curettage, cryotherapy, topical keratolytics, topical potassium hydroxide, and imiquimod.

Other viral infections: A case of vaccinia is also been reported following tattoo.[25] Marshall et al. described herpes compuctorum for herpes simplex

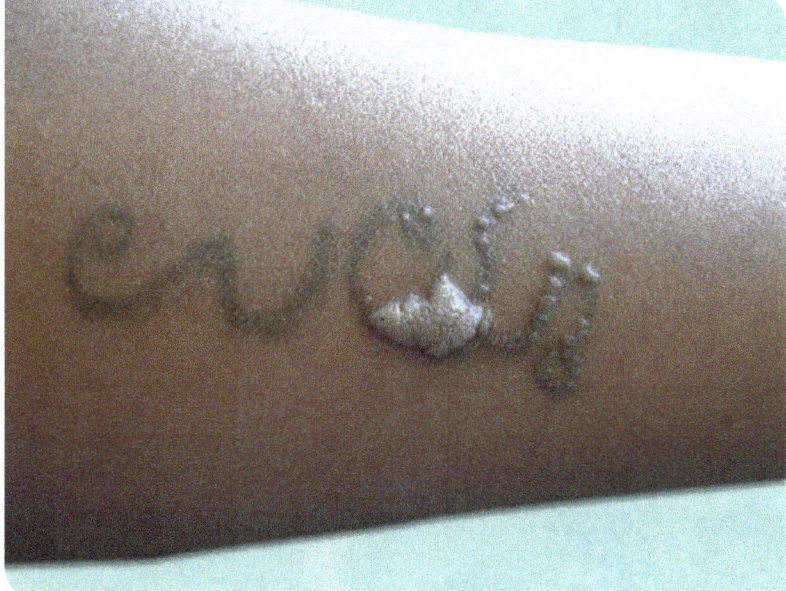

Fig. 6.7: Verruca vulgaris over tattoo.

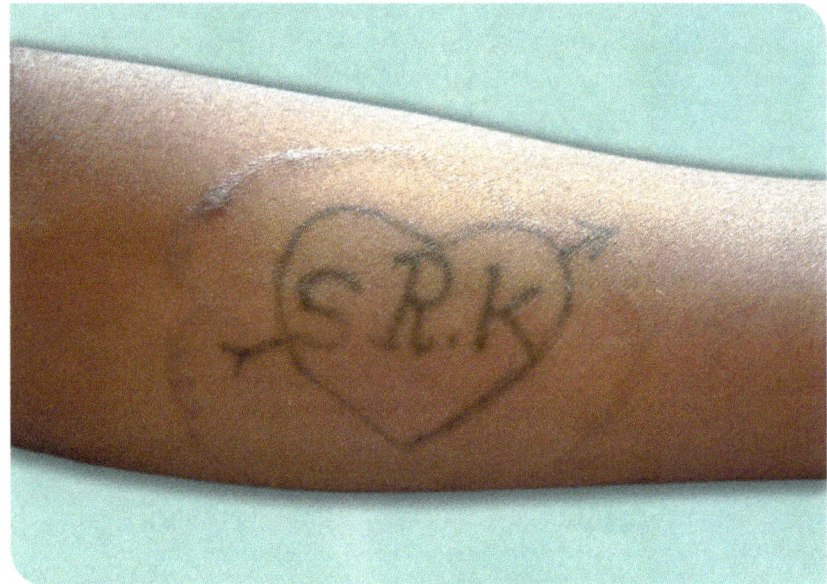

Fig. 6.8: Tinea corporis over the tattoo.

virus infection complicating tattooing.[27] Herpes infections have also reported following cosmetic lip tattooing. Rare case of herpes zoster is also reported in literature.[25]

FUNGAL INFECTIONS

Many infections secondary to mycosis like dermatophytosis (Fig. 6.8), *Aspergillus* and *Candida* have been described in literature following tattooing. Ammirati reported tinea secondary to *Trichophyton tonsurans* that occurred 2 weeks after tattooing, clinically presenting as concentric annular lesions with active vesiculopustular edges, which progressively included the entire tattoo.[28] Similarly, Oanta described tinea due to *Microsporum canis*, which occurred during the healing phase.[29] A case of zygomycosis was observed after tattooing.[30] Alexandridou et al. described a case of *Candida* endophthalmitis in a 40-year-old asplenic man after tattooing.[31] *Aspergillus fumigatus* infection was described secondary to home-made tattoo.[32]

PARASITIC INFECTIONS

Many studies have reported cases of leishmaniasis occurring within a tattoo especially in human immunodeficiency virus (HIV) patients.[33,34] On the contrary, tattooing can be used to deliver oleylphosphocholine (OlPC) formulated as liposomes to treat leishmaniasis.

> **Box 6.1:** Hypersensitivity reactions to tattoo pigments.
>
> • Eczematous
> • Lichenoid
> • Photosensitivity
> • Foreign body granuloma
> • Palisading granuloma
> • Sarcoidosis-like
> • Pseudolymphomatous reactions

Hypersensitivity Reactions to Tattoo Pigments and Dyes

Allergic reactions to tattoo pigments are uncommon following tattooing because ink pigment gets encapsulated in fibrous tissue and becomes less reactive histologically.[35] Occasionally, individual may become sensitive to ink pigment or its constituents, which may manifest in several ways (Box 6.1). Onset is highly variable, ranging from immediately to 45 years after tattooing. Ink used for tattoo differs among each artist and also its composition, exact chemistry of such formulations may be difficult to identify. Red (mercury salt), green (dichromate), blue (cobalt), yellow (cadmium) pigments, and black are commonly associated with hypersensitivity reaction. But contamination of pigments with nickel sulfate or azo dyes and quinacridon may be the culprit.[25] Although, reactions to red pigment are the most common, nuances of red like pink, orange, violet, and bordeaux are also associated with tattoo reactions.[36] Increased reactions among amateur tattoo, which was done roadside may be because of acrylic paints used by some of the artists.

Clinical features: The symptoms are nonspecific, including tenderness, swelling, asymptomatic or itchy papules or nodules, isolated pruritus, swelling, and induration. Clinically, it may present as lichenoid papules and plaques (Fig. 6.9A), eczematous dermatitis (Fig. 6.9B), verrucous lesions (Fig. 6.9C) or ulcerated plaques (Fig. 6.9D). Author has reported 50 cases of cutaneous allergic reactions among 39 patients.[37] Duration of lesions ranged from 1 month to 3 years with average duration of 7 months before appearance of allergic reaction over the tattoo. Lesions were mainly located on the upper limb. Wrist, forearm, and arms were the preferred locations of tattoo among the subjects. Red color was the common color associated with reaction, which was seen among 21 (53.9%) of 39 patients. It manifested as lichenoid papules and plaques (Fig. 6.10A), ulcerated lesions (Fig. 6.10B), scaly eczematous plaque (Fig. 6.10C), and verrucous lesion (Fig. 6.10D). Allergic reaction to black pigment was second most common seen in 13 (33.3%) patients (Fig. 6.11A). Other allergies seen are to green (5.1%) color (Fig. 6.11B) and multicolor (7.7%) (Fig. 6.11C). Ninety-six percent of reactions were among patients who underwent amateur tattooing and most of them did not know the ink used.

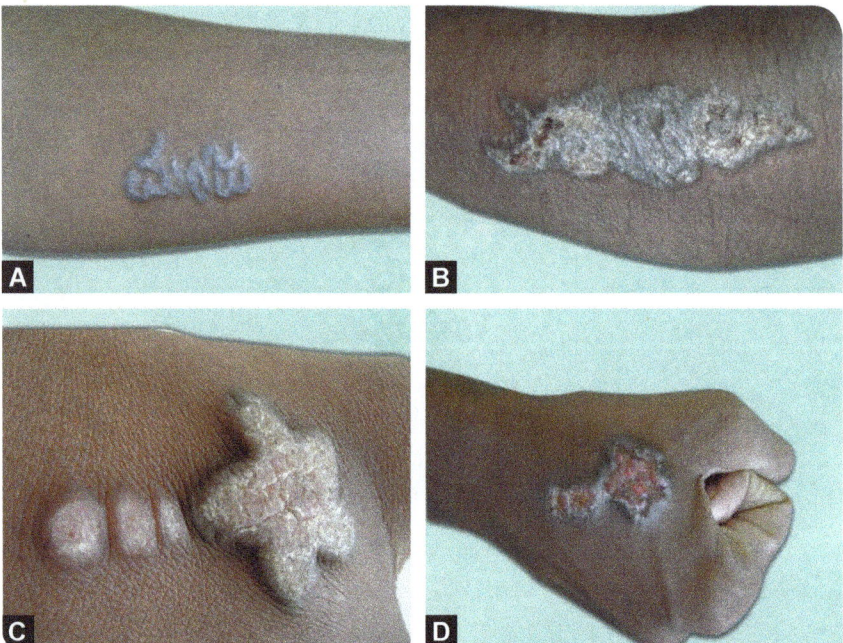

Figs. 6.9A to D: Different clinical presentation to tattoo reaction. (A) Lichenoid papules; (B) Crusted plaque—eczematous lesion; (C) Verrucous lesion; (D) Ulcerated lesion.

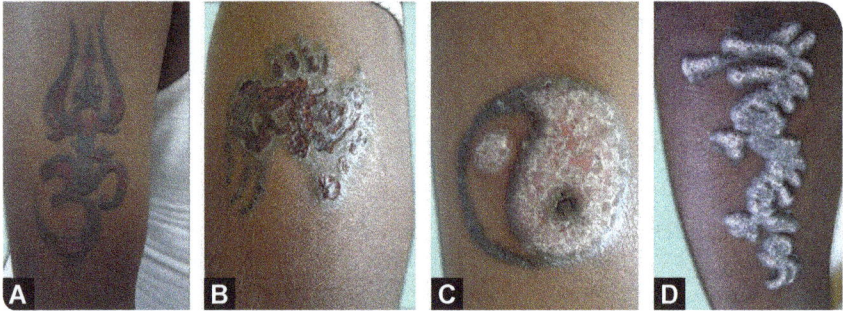

Figs. 6.10A to D: Various presentation of tattoo reaction to red color. (A) Lichenoid papules; (B) Ulcerated lesions; (C) Chronic scaly eczematous lesion; (D) Verrucous lesion.

Photosensitivity

It is one of the common allergic complications of tattoo. Sometimes, photosensitivity may be the only symptom. Sun may interact with pigments in the skin and provoke clinically significant reactions that may or may not motivate the tattooed person to seek medical advice. A "Beach study" by Carlsen on tattooed individual revealed that 52% of tattooed individuals experience one or other sun-induced reaction over tattooed area. Common

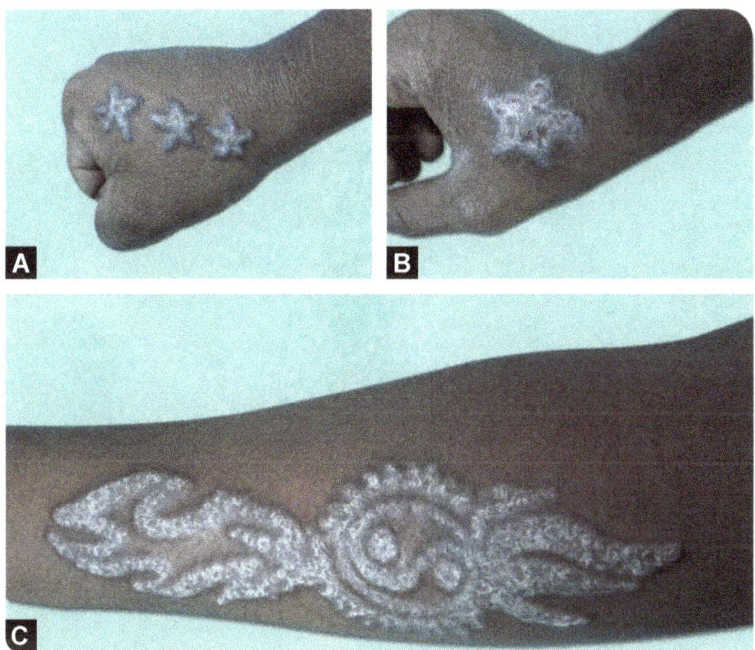

Figs. 6.11A to C: Allergic reaction to different color (A) Eczematous plaque to black pigment; (B) Elevated plaque to green ink; (C) Verrucous lesion to multicolor tattoo.

presentations were swelling, itching, stinging, pain, and redness, predominantly in black and red tattoos. Reaction may be frequent in blue tattoos, but may not be confined to one specific color or chemical entity or class of pigment. Photochemical reactions to pigment or pigment-breakdown products in situ in the skin with induction of reactive oxygen species (ROS) is presumed to be one causative mechanism. Another possible mechanism especially relevant in black may be induction of ROS due to effects of aggregation of carbon black nanoparticles.[38]

Tattoo-induced Pseudolymphoma

It is a rare complication, first described by Okun and Edelstein in 1976.[39] Pseudolymphoma is a histological diagnosis of a benign process of reactive hyperplasia of lymphocytes not meeting criteria for malignant lymphoma. The mechanism for the development of tattoo-induced pseudolymphoma is unknown. A proposed mechanism is that the pigment of the tattoo acts as an antigen, which induces the proliferation of lymphocytes, causing the localized reaction that is clinically seen.[40]

Investigations: Histopathological examination of a punch skin biopsy specimen is mandatory for the proper diagnosis. It can show lichenoid reaction (Figs. 6.12A to C), spongiotic (Figs. 6.13A and B), foreign body reaction

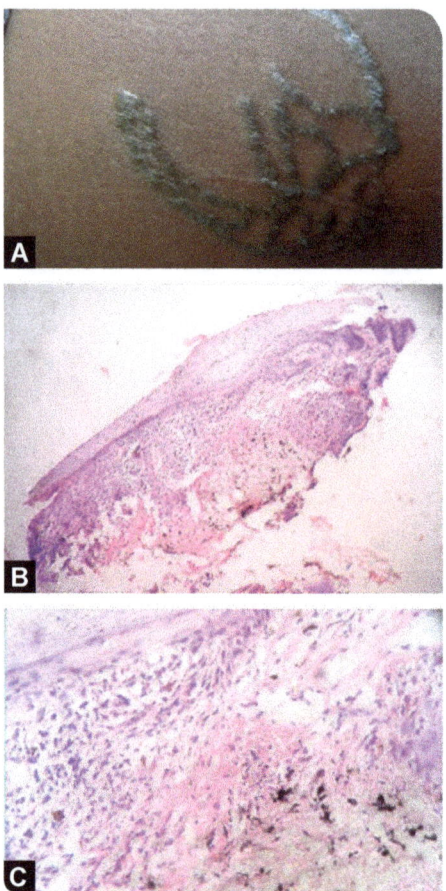

Figs. 6.12A to C: Lichenoid reaction pattern of tattoo allergy. (A) Lichenoid reaction to black pigment; (B) 100×, H and E, hyperkeratosis and parakeratosis with dense lymphocytic infiltration at dermoepidermal junction with pigment incontinence; (C) 400× H and E, lymphocytic infiltration in dermoepidermal junction.

(Figs. 6.14A to C), palisading granuloma (Figs. 6.15A to C), and sarcoidal reaction (3.3%) (Figs. 6.16A and B). Diagnostic patch testing often shows negative results may be because suitable patch test solutions are difficult to obtain owing to the low-dispersing capacities of most pigments. Tests can be performed, if the culprit ink is available and its composition is known; however, it is not always possible to reproduce the reaction induced with tattooing. Authors reported positive patch test using Fevicryl Acrylic colors,® which was culprit in amateur tattoo (Figs. 6.17A and B).[37] X-ray analysis may be performed on cutaneous biopsies and/or on the ink, but identification of the compound responsible is difficult, and it is not always possible to rule out that another unidentified compound may be responsible for the reaction.[7]

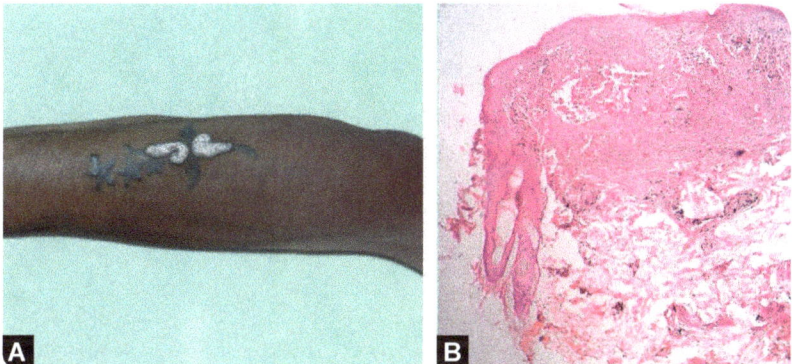

Figs. 6.13A and B: Eczematous reaction to red pigment. (A) Eczematous reaction to red pigment; (B) 400x, H and E, thinned epidermis at places with spongiosis and blister formation (filled with fluid and polymorphs) pigment deposition in epidermis with pigment incontinence at dermis and inflammatory cells infiltrate.

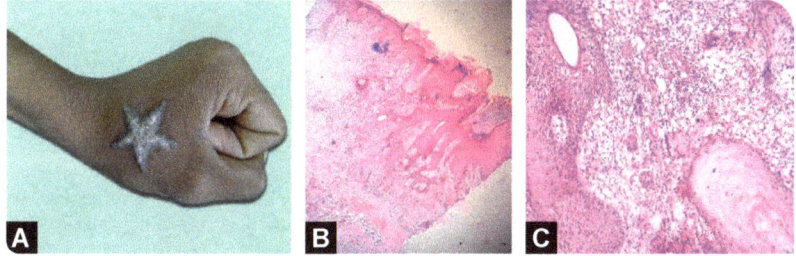

Figs. 6.14A to C: Foreign body reaction to red dye. (A) Eczematous lesion over wrist; (B) 50×, H and E, hyperkeratosis, acanthosis, follicular plugging, with foreign body reaction to pigment; (C) 400x, H and E, dense lymphocytic infiltrate, mononuclear cell infiltrate around blood vessel, foreign body like giant cells, pigment incontinence.

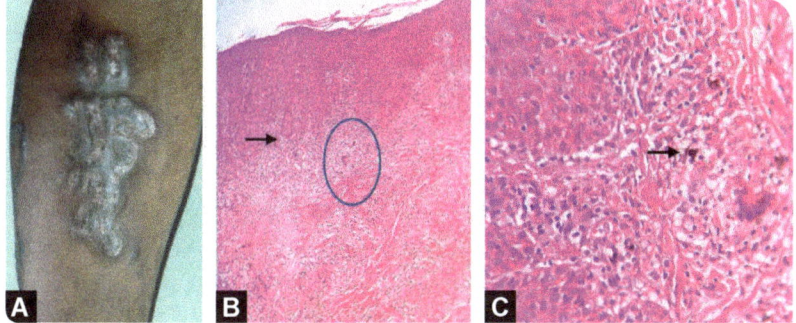

Figs. 6.15A to C: Palisading granuloma to tattoo ink. (A) Eczematous lesion over forearm; (B) 100×, H and E, palisading granuloma (Circle) in mid reticular dermis around focus of mucin deposition and incomplete collagen degeneration; (C) 400x, H and E, the granuloma consists of lymphocytes, histiocytes, and occasional giant cells and forms a semicircular palisade. Small red pigment granules (arrow) are seen at the periphery of this focus amongst histiocytes.

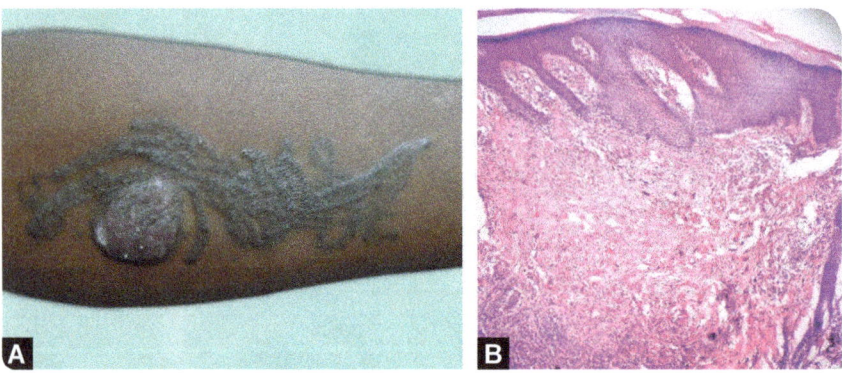

Figs. 6.16A and B: Sarcoidal reaction to multicolor dye. (A) Well-defined plaque over tattoo; (B) 400x, H and E, dense lymphocytic infiltrate with sarcoidal granuloma.

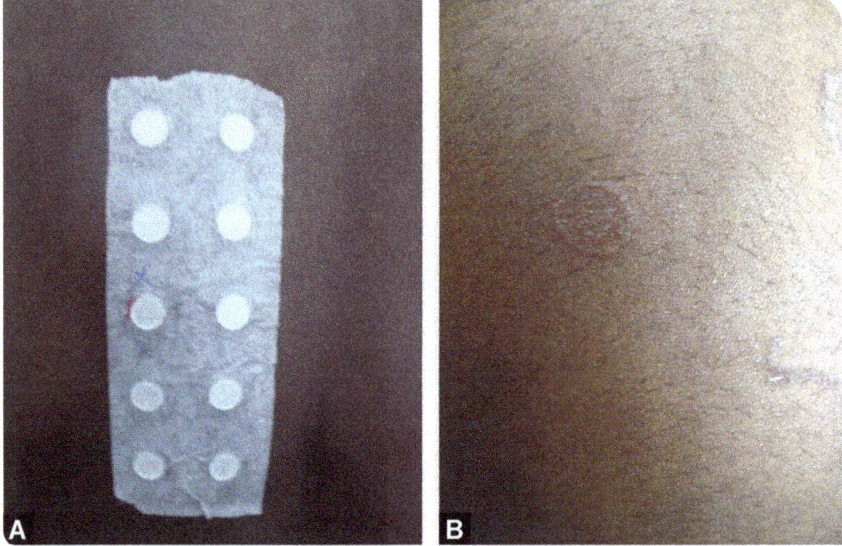

Figs. 6.17A and B: Patch test with Fevicryl® stock solution. (A) Red Paint is used for testing; (B) Positive response after 48 hours.

Treatment:[7] Treatment is often difficult and usually only temporary as long as the ink responsible is still present in the skin. Topical corticosteroids are the mainstay therapy to control exacerbation (Figs. 6.18A to C). The main problem is prompt relapse after stopping topical steroid. Intralesional corticosteroids can be administrated for resistant lesion and thick lesions. Perilesion hypo-/depigmentation is a known complication (Fig. 6.19). Topical tacrolimus or pimecrolimus are other possible treatments. If the lesion is hypertrophic, cryotherapy is also an option (Fig. 6.20). Lasers have very limited role in hypersensitivity reaction due to tattoo. Fractional CO_2 or

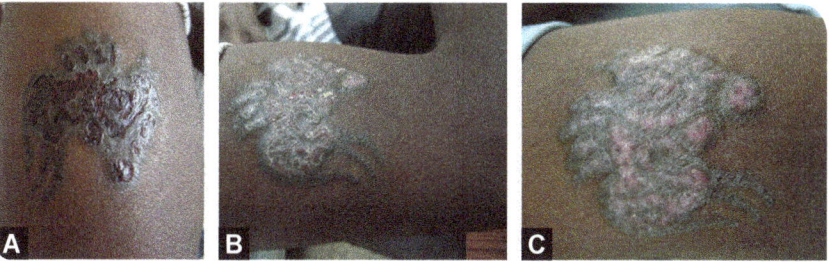

Figs. 6.18A to C: Hypersensitivity reaction to red dye treated with topical steroid.

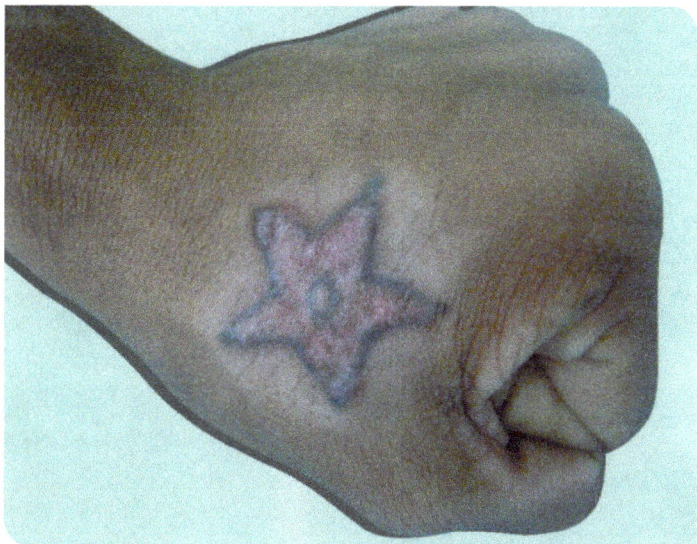

Fig. 6.19: Tattoo reaction to red color treated with intralesional steroid shows perilesional hypopigmentation.

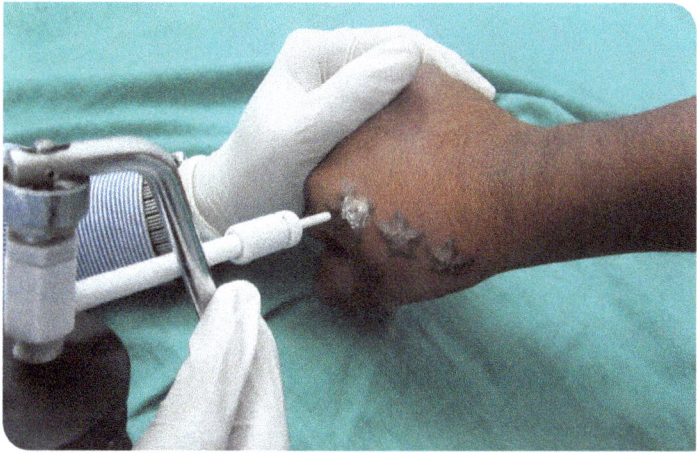

Fig. 6.20: Verrucous tattoo reaction treated with cryotherapy.

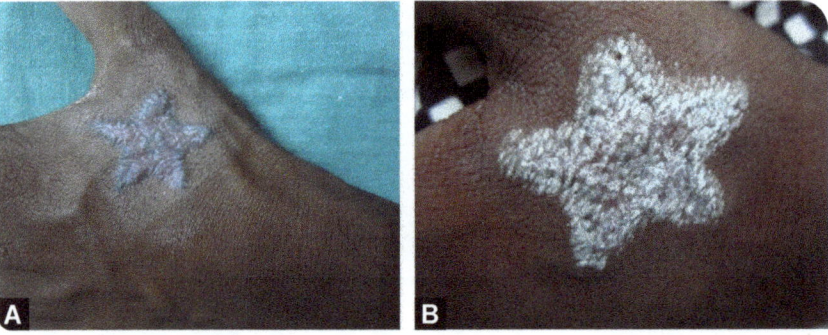

Figs. 6.21A and B: Allergy to red dye treated with 532 nm Q-switched Nd:YAG laser (immediate after laser).

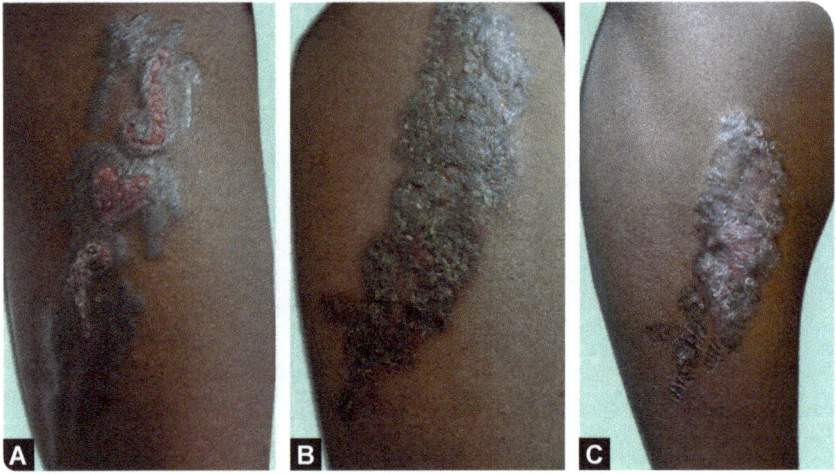

Figs. 6.22A to C: Tattoo reaction treated with fractional CO_2 followed by 532-nm Q-switched Nd:YAG laser (various stages).

Q-switched Nd:YAG laser alone or in combination may be used to hasten the clearance of the culprit pigment by breaking them (Figs. 6.21 and 6.22). Sometimes, combinations of debridement, cryotherapy, intralesional corticosteroid, and laser may be done, but decision is always on case-to-case basis and treating physician discretion (Figs. 6.23A to E). If the reaction continues, surgical excision either partial (Figs. 6.24A and B) or complete (Figs. 6.25A and B) is the treatment of choice. Excision can be elliptical, serial, or rotational flaps, or sometimes graft can be placed. Precaution should be taken when performing laser treatment of a tattoo with hypersensitivity reaction. A case of a generalized allergic reaction after CO_2 laser has been reported.[41] In authors experience, surgical excision is ideal with through irrigation of the wound site to remove finest pigment.

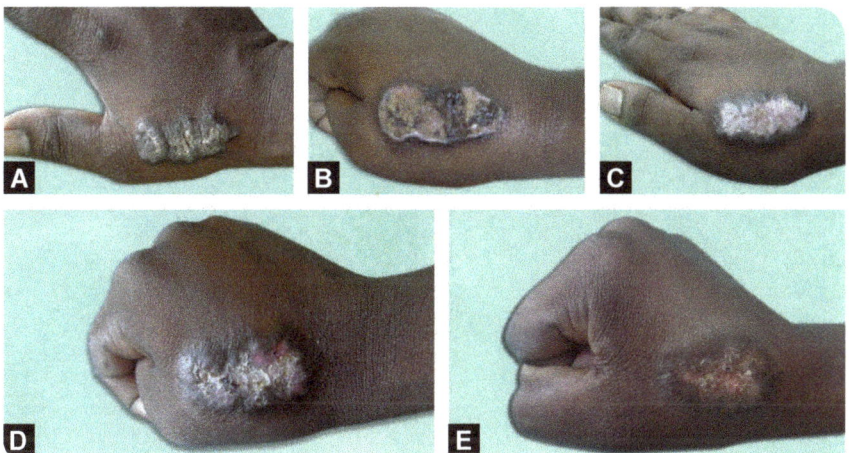

Figs. 6.23A to E: Tattoo hypersensitivity treated with multiple modalities—intralesional steroid followed by cryotherapy and debridement and resultant scar.

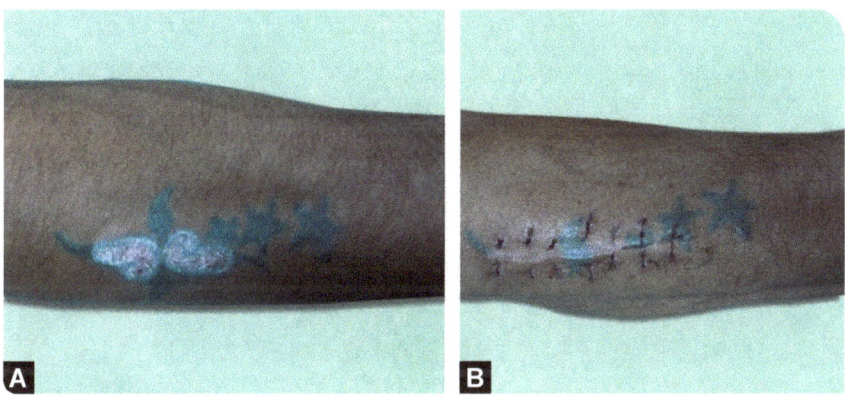

Figs. 6.24A and B: Partial excision of the abnormal portion in a patient to red pigment allergy.

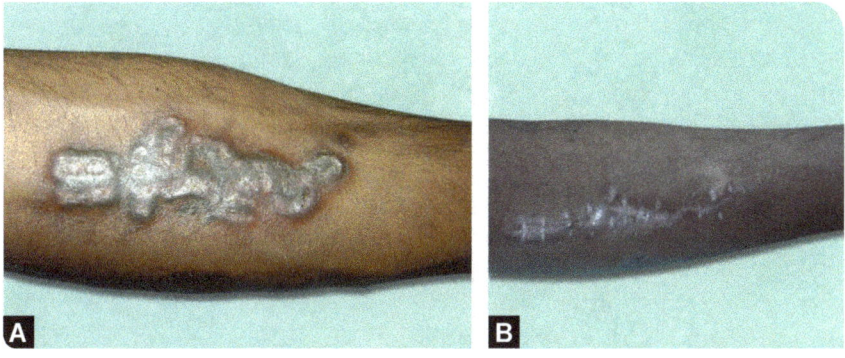

Figs. 6.25A and B: Complete excision and suturing of allergy tattoo reaction.

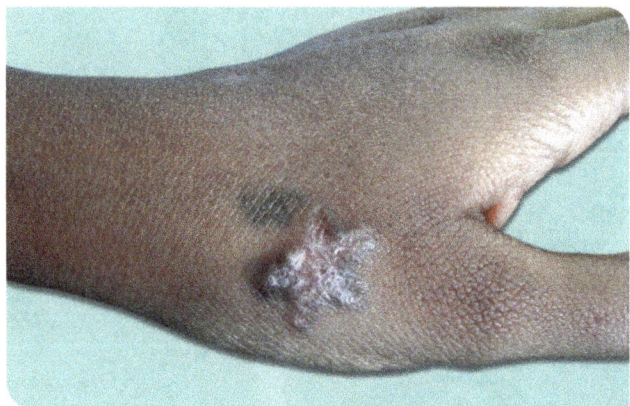

Fig. 6.26: Residual atrophic scar after prolonged waxing and waning of allergic tattoo reaction.

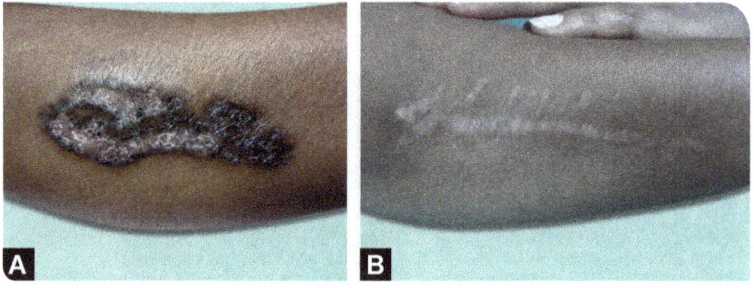

Figs. 6.27A and B: Residual scar after tattoo reaction, which was excised to remove ugly scar.

Prognosis: Hypersensitivity reactions can resolve spontaneously, remain active or wax, and wane for years. Periodic episodes of skin reactions are common, but patients seek medical attention only if the reaction becomes disabling or severe.[7] In author's experience, waxing and waning continues till the last trace of pigment is removed from the body either by macrophages or through epidermal elimination. This usually heals over the years leaving behind scar (Fig. 6.26). Sometimes, patient may seek advice for the removal of residual scar (Figs. 6.27A and B).

Prevention: Avoiding tattoo is the most ideal preventive measure. If a patient has experienced a color-specific tattoo reaction, he or she should be discouraged from getting tattooed with the same color, even if the ink brand is different. People with allergy to red pigment may opt another color tattoo with caution as potential risk of reaction to another color due to a common substance in both inks have been reported.[7] Cross-reaction with allergic manifestation at distant tattoo site due to concomitant raection to is known phenomenon (Fig. 6.28).

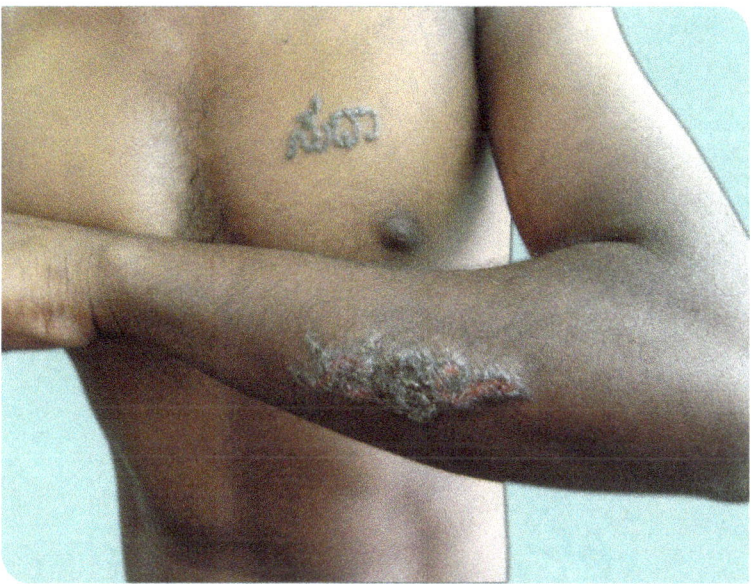

Fig. 6.28: Allergy reaction to red color on the left forearm with concomitant reaction over existing black tattoo over chest.

Table 6.4:	Skin tumors occurring on tattoos.
Benign	Traumatized nevus, seborrheic keratoses, histiocytofibroma, epidermal cysts, milia
Malignant	Eruptive or isolated keratoacanthoma, melanoma, basal cell carcinoma, squamous cell carcinoma, cutaneous lymphoma, leiomyosarcoma, dermatofibrosarcoma protuberans
Others	Pseudoepitheliomatous hyperplasia

Skin Tumors Arising on Tattoos

The potential local and systemic carcinogenic effects of tattoos and tattoo inks remain unclear. Several studies have shed light on the presence of potential carcinogenic or procarcinogenic products in tattoo inks. Many benign and malignant tumors have been described in literature associated with tattoo (Table 6.4). Numerous factors could be involved, including intradermal injection of potentially carcinogenic substances (benzapyrene in black tattoo ink), exposure to ultraviolet (UV) radiation, and genetic factors. But still debate is continuing on role of tattoos in pathogenesis of tumor.[7,42]

Pseudoepitheliomatous hyperplasia: The epidermal hyperplasia has been proposed to represent the pathway to neoplasia, as case of squamous cell carcinoma (SCC) on pseudoepitheliomatous hyperplasia (PEH).[43] It manifests as multiple verrucous papules mainly associated with red tattoos

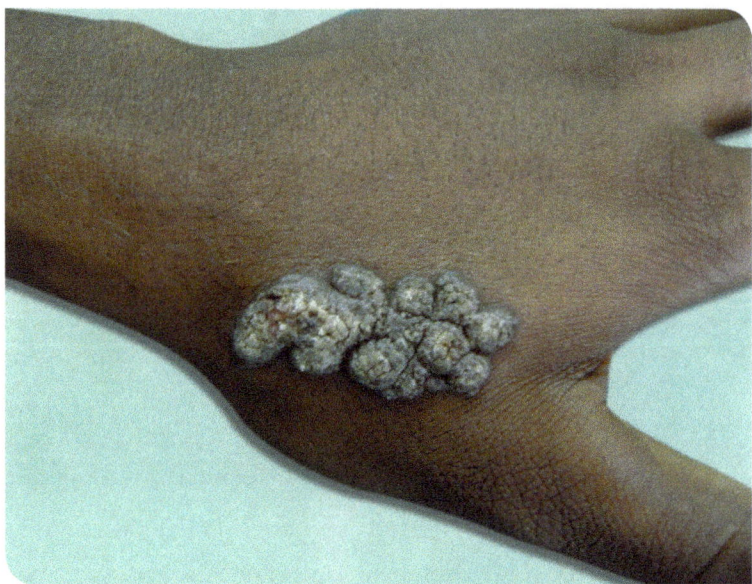

Fig. 6.29: Pseudoepitheliomatous hyperplastic reaction of tattooed area.

(Fig. 6.29). Histopathology shows prominent infundibular hyperplasia and differentiating with keratoacanthoma (KA) may be difficult. Associated lichenoid infiltration is common and marks lichenoid reaction pattern. Treatment options include excision and topical or injected corticosteroids.[44,45]

Benign tumors: Sudden clinical change may be triggered after tattooing over the benign nevi and may warrant further investigations to distinguish between a traumatized nevus and malignant degeneration. Benign cases of seborrheic keratosis, histiocytofibroma, epidermal cysts, and milia have been reported.[46]

Malignant Tumors

Keratoacanthoma: It is a common keratinizing squamous cell neoplasm of unknown origin characterized by rapid growth and spontaneous involution. Clinically presents as isolated, single lesions over sun-exposed areas, but rarely can be multiple and eruptive but known to occur in initial post-tattoo period in contrast to SCC. Histopathology shows strands and nodules of atypical squamous cells with mitotic activity and cellular atypia that become less prominent as the neoplasms progress into the maturation phase. Therapy includes excision, radiotherapy, cryotherapy, laser therapy, systemic agents like cyclophosphamide and retinoids, intralesional methotrexate, bleomycin, 5-fluorouracil, steroids, and topical agents, such as imiquimod alone or in combination with retinoic acid.[47]

Table 6.5: Localization of skin disorders to tattoos.

Sarcoidosis	Perforating dermatosis
Psoriasis	Granuloma annulare
Discoid lupus	Morphea
Subacute lupus	Postinflammatory scleroderma-like reaction
Cutaneous vasculitis	Pyoderma gangrenosum
Darier's disease	Lichen planus
Vitiligo	Lichen sclerosus and atrophicus
Keloid	
Hypertrophic scar	

Squamous cell carcinoma: It is an unusual reaction that can occur in tattoos. Clinical diagnosis can be challenging as differential diagnoses include skin alterations based on allergic reactions, PEH, and KAs. Wide excision is the treatment.

Melanoma: Melanoma can develop within tattoos. Recognition of melanoma over tattooed areas can be difficult by the presence of surrounding pigment, which may mimic melanin pigment. Also, under microscopy, macrophages laden with tattoo pigment can appear similar to areas of regression in melanoma. Tattoo pigment is taken up by dermal macrophages and delivered to draining lymph nodes, potentially misleading surgeons and pathologists in the analysis of sentinel lymph nodes.[48]

Many studies have described development of basal cell carcinomas in a tattoo.[49,50] Lee et al. reported basal cell carcinoma in a tattooed eyebrow.[51]

Localization of Skin Disorders to Tattoos

Tattoo-related complications at the site of tattooing are common (Table 6.5). Post-tattoo keloid and hypertrophic scarring (Fig. 6.30) are common entities.

Tattoo sarcoidosis is a known entity though uncommon. Many reports of sarcoidosis in both cosmetic and amateur tattoo have been reported. Reactions in cosmetic tattoos and relating to sarcoidosis have been reported as early as 1952. The cause of sarcoidal reactions in tattoos remains unknown. This finding may be a specific cutaneous manifestation of sarcoidosis in which the pigment in tattoos acts as a nidus for granuloma formation; such reactions may be the only manifestation of cutaneous sarcoidosis. Alternatively, the systemic spread of the tattoo pigment could cause a reaction in other sites, simulating systemic sarcoidosis. However, if other clinical features are present such as uveitis or pulmonary involvement, the possibility of systemic sarcoidosis should be considered.[52-54]

Psoriasis is a common papulosquamous condition and occurrence of psoriatic lesion over the tattooed areas is well-described phenomenon

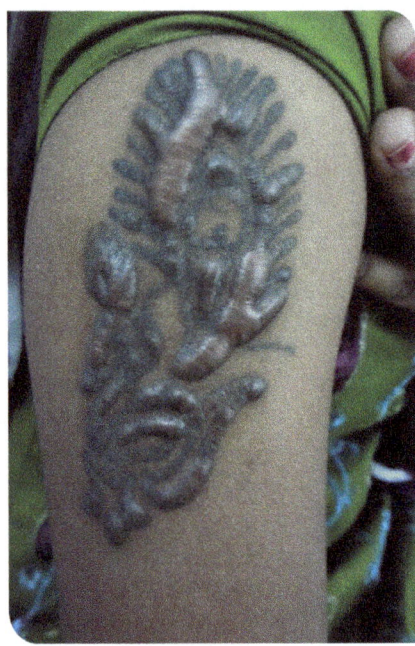

Fig. 6.30: Hypertrophic scar following tattooing.

secondary to Koebnerization. Ghorpade described unusual case where patient had no previous personnel or family history of psoriasis but developed psoriatic lesion confined to the tattooed areas after tattooing.[55] Similar case who developed psoriatic arthritis later also has been described.[56]

Chronic discoid lupus and subacute cutaneous lupus lesions have been reported on tattoos, either in an isolated fashion or associated with other localization.[6,57,58] Lichen planus on tattoo may be an isolated phenomenon where it represents true hypersensitivity reaction to tattoo granules. Otherwise, it can be a manifestation of generalized lichen planus. Difficulty arises in differentiating case of generalized lichenoid eruption secondary to tattoo with true lichen planus.[7]

Tattooing can lead to koebnerization in patients with vitiligo (Fig. 6.31) and pyoderma gangrenosum. A case of xerotic eczema was reported on tattoo (Fig. 6.32). Other skin disorders localizing at the tattoo site are enumerated in Table 6.5.

Interference with Medical Devices and Imaging Results Disturbance[7]

Tattoo may cause interference with many investigations (Box 6.2). Dermoscopy evaluation to rule out melanoma may be difficult, if the lesion is tattooed. Others interferences are described in Box 6.2.

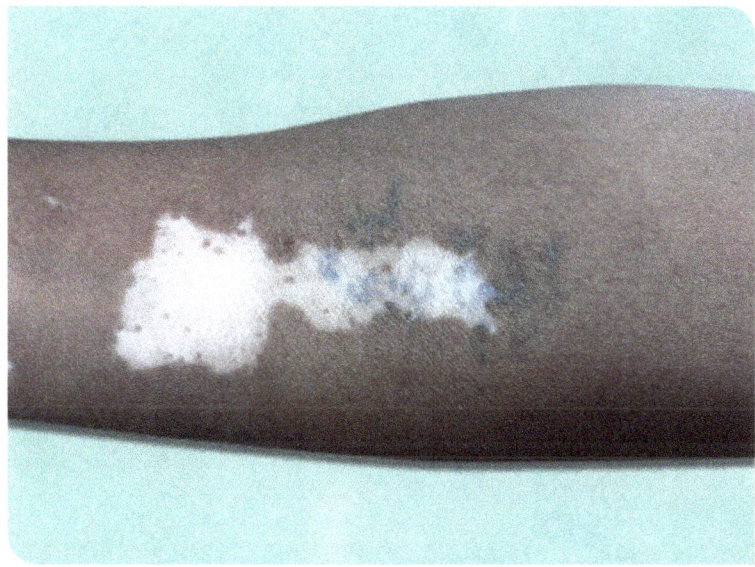

Fig. 6.31: Vitiligo over tattoo leading to fading of color.

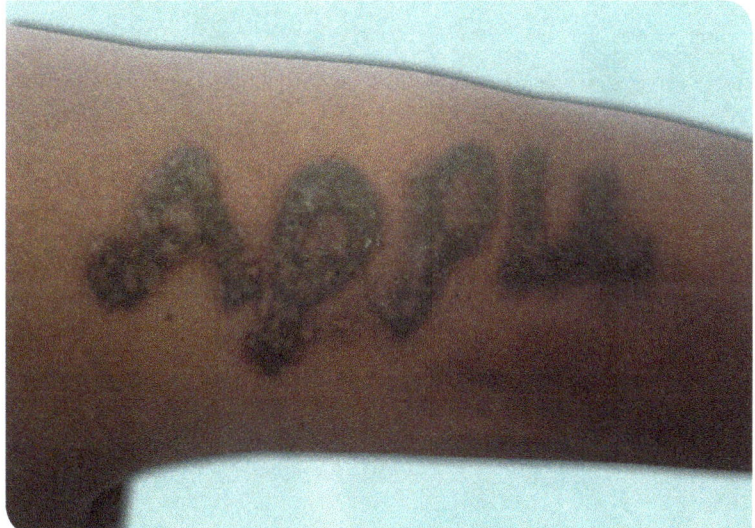

Fig. 6.32: Xerotic eczema over the tattoo.

Miscellaneous Complications

Color fading (Fig. 6.33) and color changing in a tattoo is depressing for the patient. This can happen with both medical and decorative tattoo. Inherent property of pigment, migration of tattoo, sunlight, and other factors may be responsible.

- Disturbance of dermoscopy examination on tattooed areas
- Tingling/burning sensations during NMR (nuclear magnetic resonance) examination
- False-positive marker uptake on lymph nodes on positron emission tomography (PET)-scan false-positive sentinel lymph node, axillary lymph node calcifications on mammography
- Interference with plethysmograph sensor especially wrist tattoo

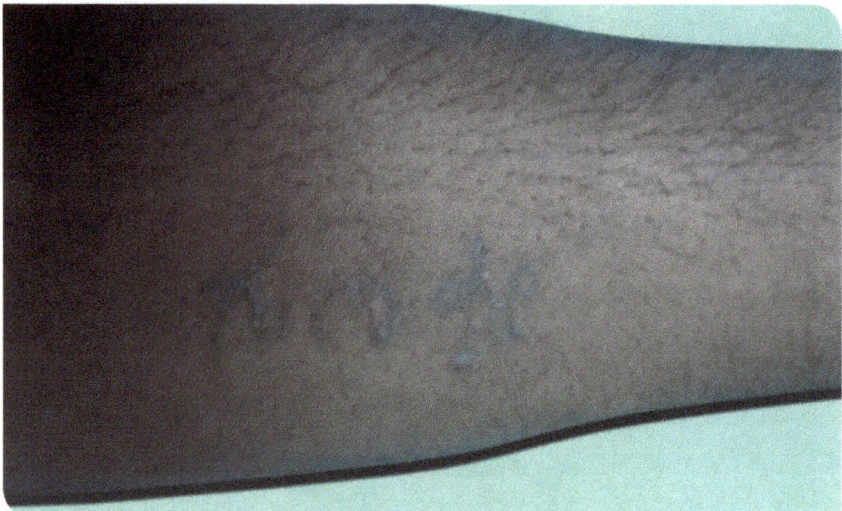

Fig. 6.33: Fading of amateur tattoo over the period.

Psychosocial Complications

The main complication of tattooing is regret. This is true with impulse tattoo or group tattoo (Figs. 6.34A to C). Psychosocial risks exist when tattooed person feels disappointment or low self-esteem, or suffers embarrassment because they are not satisfied with the product or are distressed by the public's or their family's response to the tattoo, which is common with adolescent. Removal of tattoo is also difficult leading to frustration.

Complications of Tattoo Removal

Tattoo removal is a very cumbersome procedure, and it may not always be successful. Also, complications are common with laser tattoo removal (Table 6.6). Details of complications and its prevention are included in chapter on laser tattoo removal.

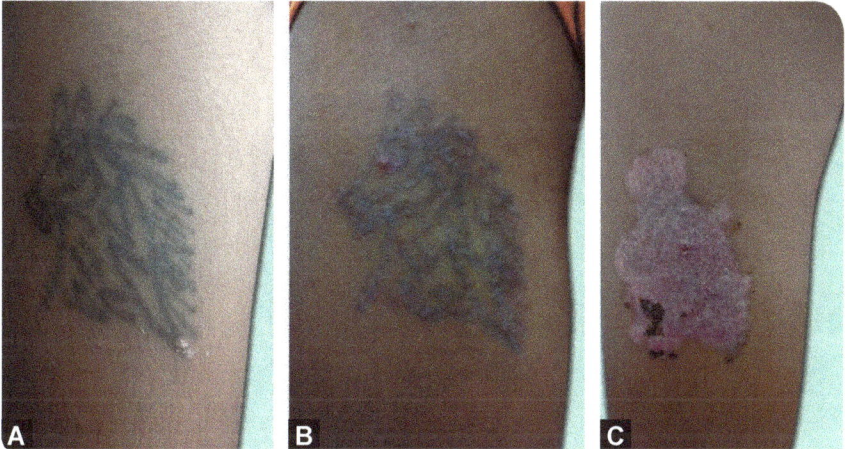

Figs. 6.34A to C: A case of tattoo over left in an army aspirate who sought laser tattoo removal but ended up burning the lesion in order to get quick results.

Table 6.6: Complications of tattoo removal.[1]	
Immediate	Pain, blisters, crusting, pinpoint hemorrhage
Delayed	Hyperpigmentation, hypopigmentation, leukotrichia, paradoxical darkening, residual tattoos, textural changes and scarring, local or generalized reaction

Extracutaneous Complications

Extracutaneous complication secondary to tattooing can be either systemic allergic reaction or blood-borne infections (BBV) (*see* Fig. 6.1), which are secondary to inoculation but not confined to tattooed area (Flowchart 6.1).

Anaphylaxis

Two reports of life-threatening anaphylactic reactions, immediately after permanent tattooing, while in tattoo parlor have been reported.[59,60] In first case, 30-year-old atopic women who developed anaphylaxis in her 3rd or 4th tattoo.[60] Second case was a 59-year-old male who developed anaphylaxis 5 hours after tattooing. Main allergen identified was formaldehyde, a known preservative used in cosmetic. While formaldehyde is unable to penetrate through an intact epidermal barrier made of cornified keratinocytes (i.e. stratum corneum), direct injection into living and vascularized dermal tissue as in case with tattooing, may result in immediate systemic bioavailability leading to anaphylaxis.[61] Clinicians should be alert to the potential capacity of tattoo inks to act as triggers of systemic anaphylaxis.

Flowchart 6.1: Extracutaneous complications.

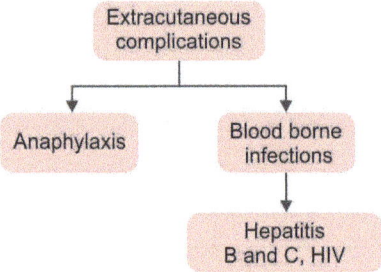

Blood-borne Infections

Tattoos are associated with BBV infections that result from viruses such as the hepatitis B virus (HBV), the hepatitis C virus (HCV), and the HIV. Abiona's study revealed that tattoos and body-piercings in prison were important risk factors associated with the transmission of BBV infections.[62] Cross-infections due to sharing of contaminated needles, ink-wells, or the tattooists' hands or cloth in setting like unregulated establishments, on the streets, in jails, and in ritual ceremonies/mela/fare.

A systemic and meta-analysis comprising of 124 studies indicated a strong association between tattooing and the risk of hepatitis and concluded that tattoo is a strong risk factor for transmission of hepatitis C for two reasons:[63]

1. Several studies have reported an association between tattooing and other infections including HIV, hepatitis B, leprosy, and MRSA.
2. Some studies have shown that the risk of hepatitis infection increases with the increase in the surface area covered by a tattoo, as well as the number of tattoos received by an individual.

An another systematic review and meta-analysis by Jafari et al. on 41 observational studies observed association of tattooing with hepatitis B infection and demonstrated strongest association between tattooing and risk of hepatitis B among populations involved in high-risk behaviors.[64]

There is paucity of data for transmission of HIV through tattoo,[65,66] but theoretically it is possible. HIV has been shown to remain infectious in aqueous solutions at room temperature for up to 15 days[67] and pigmented solutions, because they are relatively inert, may also support the virus.[65] Thus, tattooing gun, needles, pigment wells, and swab may be a potential source of contamination for BBV infectious diseases. Also, a systematic review published in 2001 found that tattoos are more commonly found among HIV-positive individuals than in control groups or the general population.[66] Two cases of HIV infection in the US likely to have been acquired by tattooing within prison was reported by Doll.[68]

Table 6.7: Complications of henna tattoo.	
Allergic	• Type I hypersensitivity reaction like sneezing, conjunctivitis, running nose, dry cough, dyspnea, swelling of the face, or generalized urticaria • Type IV hypersensitivity reaction in the form of contact allergic reaction
Nonallergic	Hemolysis in G6PD deficiency children, problems with peripheral venous cannulation

(G6PD: Glucose-6-phosphatase dehydrogenase).

Complications of Temporary Tattoo

Temporary henna tattoos have become increasingly widespread among children and young people, especially in holiday spots in recent years. As compared to permanent henna tattoo, temporary tattooing is painless, cheap, can be applied anywhere, lasts for days, is fun to decorate, easy to remove, and carries no risk of infections.[69] It has been used as a dye for the skin, hair, and nails for over 4,000 years, and as an expression of body art, especially in Islamic and Hindu cultures in the Arab, African, and Indian world.[70] With increased popularity, there are report of progressive increase in reactions to henna and black henna tattoo.

Henna Tattoo

Red henna appears to be generally safe but there are many reports of allergic and nonallergic complications (Table 6.7). Avoidance of culprit agent is the rule. Topical and systemic steroid will help in the treatment.

Temporary Black Henna Tattoo

Black henna is the combination of henna proper and p-Phenylenediamine (PPD). PPD is added to henna to accelerate the dyeing and drying process (to only 30 minutes), to strengthen and darken the color, to enhance the design pattern of the tattoo, and to make the tattoo last longer. These tattoos stain the skin black, and have the appearance of a real tattoo. Most of the complications are due to PPD component in black henna (Table 6.8). Contact dermatitis is the most common complication. Black henna tattoos will induce contact allergy to its ingredient PPD at an estimated frequency of 2.5%. Once sensitized, the patients may experience allergic contact dermatitis from the use of hair dyes containing PPD (Figs. 6.35 and 6.36). There are often cross-reactions to other hair dyes, dyes used in textiles, local anesthetics, and rubber chemicals. The diagnosis is easy to suspect on the basis of

Table 6.8: Complications of temporary black henna tattoo.[70]	
Cutaneous	• Contact dermatitis—allergic contact dermatitis, hand dermatitis, lichenoid contact dermatitis, erythema multiforme-like contact dermatitis • Cross-sensitization to other dye • Localized hypertrichosis • Second-degree chemical burn • Leukoderma • Hyperpigmentation • Hypertrophic or keloid scar
Systemic	• Anaphylaxis • Cutaneous vasculitis • Crescentic rapidly progressive glomerulonephritis • Sweet syndrome

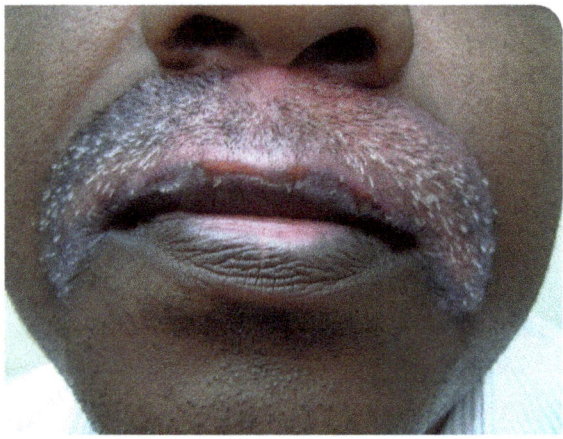

Fig. 6.35: Allergic contact dermatitis of beard area secondary to black henna.

the clinical picture, and can be confirmed by a positive patch test reaction to PPD. Increased popularity of henna as a "safe alternative" may increase the use of black henna tattoos without any legislation to control its use. Thus, authorities in every country should monitor to minimize the damage and to discourage its use.

CONCLUSION

Disadvantages of tattooing (Box 6.3) always overweigh its advantages and also health risks are growing with advent of newer dyes. Infections and hypersensitivity reaction, are on the rise. Proper health education at schools and college, can stop this growing menace. Also proper regulation and legislation are the need of the hour.

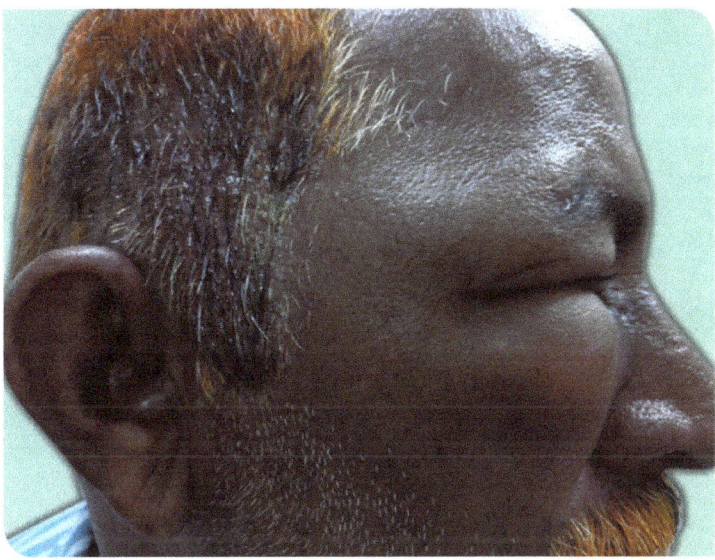

Fig. 6.36: Allergic contact dermatitis of scalp secondary to black henna hair dye in a person using henna, who wanted to try black hair dye.

Box 6.3: Summary of cutaneous complications of tattoos.[7]

Acute inflammatory reaction: Pain, bleeding, purpura/hematoma, crusts, inflammation, contact dermatitis, blue-foot/tattoo blow-out, improper healing with scars.

Infections occurring on tattoos:
Bacterial infections:
- *Pyogenic infections*: Folliculitis, furunculosis, erysipelas, necrotizing fasciitis, gangrene
- *Nonpyogenic infections*: Atypical mycobacteria, inoculation leprosy, inoculation tuberculosis, inoculation syphilis, tetanus
- *Viral infections*: Viral wart (verruca vulgaris), molluscum contagiosum, Herpes simplex (Herpes compunctorum), Herpes zoster
- *Fungal*: Tinea, Sporotrichosis, Zygomycosis, Blastomycosis, Mycetoma, Aspergillus fumigatus
- *Parasitic*: Leishmaniasis.

Hypersensitivity reactions to tattoo pigments: Eczematous, lichenoid, photosensitivity, foreign body granuloma, palisading granuloma, sarcoidosis-like and pseudolymphomatous reactions.

Tumors occurring on tattoo:
- *Benign*: Traumatized nevus, seborrheic keratoses, histiocytofibroma, epidermal cysts, milia
- *Malignant*: Eruptive or isolated keratoacanthoma, melanoma, basal cell carcinoma, squamous cell carcinoma, cutaneous lymphoma, leiomyosarcoma, dermatofibrosarcoma protuberans
- *Others*: Pseudoepitheliomatous hyperplasia

Contd...

Contd...

Localization of skin disorders: Sarcoidosis, psoriasis, discoid lupus, subacute lupus, cutaneous vasculitis, Darier's disease, vitiligo, keloid, hypertrophic scar, lichen planus, lichen sclerosus and atrophicus, perforating dermatosis (perforating collagenosis, perforating granuloma annulare), granuloma annulare, morphea, postinflammatory scleroderma-like reaction, pyoderma gangrenosum.

Interference with medical devices and imaging results disturbance: Disturbance of dermoscopy examination on tattooed areas, keloid/burn after laser therapy, tingling/burning sensations during NMR (nuclear magnetic resonance) examination, false-positive marker uptake on lymph nodes on positron emission tomography (PET)-scan, false-positive sentinel lymph node, axillary lymph node calcifications on mammography, interference with plethysmograph sensor especially wrist tattoo.

Miscellaneous complications: Color fading, color changing

Psychosocial complications

Complications of tattoo removal:

Immediate: Pain, blisters, crusting, pinpoint hemorrhage

Delayed: Hyperpigmentation, hypopigmentation, leukotrichia, paradoxical darkening, residual tattoos, textural changes and scarring, Local allergic reactions

---

REFERENCES

1. Khunger N, Molpariya A, Khunger A. Complications of tattoos and tattoo removal: Stop and think before you ink. J Cutan Aesthet Surg. 2015;8:30-6.
2. Laumann AE, Derik AJ. Tattoos and body piercings in the United States: a national data set. J Am Acad Dermatol. 2006;55:413.
3. Braverman S. (2012). One in five U.S. adults now has a tattoo. New York: Harris Interactive, 2012. [online] Available from http://www.theharrispoll.com/health-life/One_in_Five_U_S__Adults_Now_Has_a_Tattoo.pdf. [Accessed April, 2017].
4. European commission: JRC technical reports. Safety of tattoos and permanent make-up State of play and trends in tattoo practices. Report on Work Package 2 Administrative Arrangement N. 2014-33617 Analysis conducted on behalf of DG JUST, 2015. EUR 27528 EN ISBN 978-92-79-52789-0 (PDF); doi:10.2788/924128.
5. Klugl I, Hiller KA, Landthaler M, et al. Incidence of health problems-associated with tattooed skin: a nation-wide survey in German-speaking countries. Dermatology. 2010;221:43-50.
6. Kazandjieva J, Tsankov N. Tattoos: dermatological complications. Clin Dermatol. 2007;25:375.
7. Kluger N. Cutaneous complications related to tattooing. Forum for Nord Derm Ven. 2011;2:43-7.
8. Sperry K. Tattoos and tattooing. Part II: Gross pathology, histopathology, medical complications, and applications. Am J Forensic Med Pathol. 1992;13:7-17.
9. Kluger N, Plantier F, Moguelet P, et al. Tattoos: Natural history and histopathology of cutaneous reactions. Ann Dermatol Venereol. 2011;138:146-54, quiz 144-5.
10. Laux P, Tralau T, Tentschert J, et al. A medical-toxicological view of tattooing. Lancet. 2016;387:395-402.

11. Kazandjieva J, Tsankov N. Tattoos: dermatological complications. Clin Dermatol. 2007;25:375-82.
12. Liszewski W, Kream E, Helland S, et al. The demographics and rates of tattoo complications, regret, and unsafe tattooing practices: a cross-sectional study. Dermatol Surg. 2015;41:1283-9.
13. Dieckmann R, Boone I, O Brockmann S, et al. The risk of bacterial infection after tattooing: a systematic review of the Literature. Deutsches Ärzteblatt International. 2016;113:665-71.
14. Serup J, Hutton Carlsen K, Sepehri M. Tattoo complaints and complications: diagnosis and clinical spectrum. Curr Probl Dermatol. 2015;48:48-60.
15. Messahel A, Musgrove B. Infective complications of tattooing and skin piercing. J Infect Public Health. 2009;2:7-13.
16. Conaglen PD, Laurenson IF, Sergeant A, et al. Systematic review of tattoo-associated skin infection with rapidly growing mycobacteria and public health investigation of a cluster in Scotland, 2010. Euro Surveill. 2013;18:20553.
17. Horney DA, Gaither JM, Lauer R, et al. Cutaneous inoculation tuberculosis secondary to 'jailhouse tattooing'. Arch Dermatol. 1985;121:648-50.
18. Dhawan AK, Pandhi D, Wadhwa N, et al. Tattoo inoculation lupus vulgaris in two brothers. Indian J Dermatol Venereol Leprol. 2015;81:516-8.
19. Ghorpade A. Tattoo inoculation lupus vulgaris in two Indian ladies. J Eur Acad Dermatol Venereol. 2006;20:476-7.
20. Lowe J, Chatiirjee SN. Scarification tattooing, etc., in relation to leprous lesions in the skin. Lepr India. 1939;11:14-8.
21. Ghorpade A. Inoculation (tattoo) leprosy: a report of 31 cases. J Eur Acad Dermatol Venereol. 2002;16:494-9.
22. Ghorpade A. Reactional tattoo inoculation borderline tuberculoid leprosy with oedematous tattoos. Lepr Rev. 2004;75:91-4.
23. Long G, Rickman L. Infectious complications of tattoos. Clin Infect Dis.1994;18: 610-9.
24. Yuan J, Li W, Xia Z, et al. Secondary syphilis presenting in a red tattoo. Eur J Dermatol. 2010;20:544-5.
25. Health Canada Report. Infection prevention and control practices for personal services: tattooing, ear/bodypiercing, and electrolysis. Ontario, Canada: Laboratory Centre for Disease Control, Bureau of Infectious Diseases; 1999.
26. Foulds IS. Molluscum contagiosum: an unusual complication of tattooing. Br Med J. 1982;285:607.
27. Marshall CS, Murphy F, Mc Carthy SE. Herpes compunctorum: Cutaneous herpes simplex virus infection complicating tattooing. Med J Aust. 2007;187:598.
28. Ammirati CT. What is your diagnosis? Tinea in tattoo. Cutis. 2004;73:228-32.
29. Oanţă A, Irimie M. Tinea on a tattoo. Acta Dermatovenerol Croat. 2016;24:223-4.
30. Parker C, Kaminski G, Hill D. Zygomycosis in a tattoo, caused by Saksenaea vasiformis. Australas J Dermatol. 1986;27:107-11.
31. Alexandridou A, Reginald AY, Stavrou P, et al. Candida endophthalmitis after tattooing in an asplenic patient. Arch Ophthalmol. 2002;120:518-9.
32. Kluger N, Saarinen K. Aspergillus fumigatus infection on a home-made tattoo. Br J Dermatol. 2014;170:1373-5.
33. Garcia-Lazaro M, Villar C, Natera C, et al. Sobreelevacion de tauaje en unpaciente infectado por el virus de la inmunodeficiencia humana. Enferm Infecc Microbiol Clin. 2009;27:602-4.
34. Bosch RJ, Rodrigo AB, Sa´nchez P, et al. Presence of Leishmania organisms in specific and non-specific skin lesions in HIV-infected individuals with visceral leishmaniasis. Int J Dermatol. 2002;41:670-5.

35. Kilmer SL. Laser treatment of tattoos. Dermatol Clin. 1997;15:409-17.
36. Aberer W, Snauwaert JE, Render UM. Allergic reaction to pigments and metals. In: Christa De Cuyper (Ed). Dermatologic complications with body art: Tattoos, piercings and permanent makeup, 1st edition. Belgium: Springer link; 2010. Pp. 66-73.
37. Shashikumar BM, Harish MR, Shwetha B, et al. Hypersensitive reaction to tattoos: A growing menace in rural India. Indian J Dermatol. 2017 forthcoming.
38. Hutton Carlsen K, Serup J. Photosensitivity and photodynamic events in black, red and blue tattoos are common: A 'Beach Study, J Eur Acad Dermatol Venereol. 2014;28:231-7.
39. Okun MR, Edelstein LM. Gross and Microscopic Pathology of the Skin. Boston, MA: Dermatopathology Foundation Press; 1976.
40. Kuo WE, Richwine EE, Sheehan DJ. Pseudolymphomatous and lichenoid reaction to a red tattoo: A case report. Cutis. 2011;87:89-92.
41. Zemtsov A, Wilson L. CO_2 laser treatment causes local tattoo allergic reaction to become generalized. Acta Derm Venereol. 1997;77:497.
42. Kluger N, Phan A, Debarbieux S, et al. Skin Cancers Arising in Tattoos: Coincidental or Not? Dermatology. 2008;217:219-21.
43. Kossard S, Thompson C, Duncan GM. Hypertrophic lichen planus-like reactions combined with infundibulocystic hyperplasia: pathway to neoplasia. Arch Dermatol. 2004;140:1262-7.
44. Goldberg HI. Mercurial reaction in a tattoo. Can Med Assoc J. 1959;80:203-4.
45. Kazlouskaya V, Junkins-Hopkins JM. Pseudoepitheliomatous Hyperplasia in a Red Pigment Tattoo: A Separate Entity or Hypertrophic Lichen Planus-like Reaction? J Clin Aesth Dermatol. 2015;8:48-52.
46. Kluger N. Cutaneous complications related to permanent decorative tattooing. Expert Rev Clin Immunol. 2010;6:363-71.
47. Vitiello M, Echeverria B, Romanelli P, et al. Multiple eruptive keratoacanthomas arising in a tattoo. J Clin Aesth Dermatol. 2010;3:54-5.
48. Paprottka FJ, Bontikous S, Lohmeyer JA, et al. Squamous-cell carcinoma arises in red parts of multicolored tattoo within months. Plast Reconstr Surg Glob Open. 2014;2:e114.
49. Bashir AH. Basal cell carcinoma in tattoos: report of two cases. Br J Plast Surg. 1976;29:288-90.
50. Earley MJ. Basal cell carcinoma arising in tattoos: a clinical report of two cases. Br J Plast Surg. 1983;36:258-9.
51. Lee JS, Park J, Kim SM, et al. Basal cell carcinoma arising in a tattooed eyebrow. Ann Dermatol. 2009;21:281-4.
52. Ali SM, Gilliam A, Brodell R. Sarcoidosis appearing in a tattoo. J Cutan Med Surg. 2008;12:43-8.
53. Papageorgiou PP, Hongcharu W, Chu AC. Systemic sarcoidosis presenting with multiple tattoo granulomas and an extra-tattoo cutaneous granuloma. J Eur Acad Dermatol Venereol. 1999;12:51-3.
54. Rorsman H, Brehmer-Anderson E, Dahlquist I, et al. Tattoo granuloma and uveitis. Lancet. 1969;2:27-8.
55. Ghorpade A. Tattoo-induced psoriasis. Int J Dermatol. 2015;54:1180-2.
56. Punzi L, Rizzi E, Pianon M, et al. Tattooing-induced psoriasis and psoriatic arthritis. Br J Rheumatol. 1977;36:1129-36.
57. Beerman H, Lane RA. Tattoo; a survey of some of the literature concerning the medical complications of tattooing. Am J Med Sci. 1954;227:444-64.

58. Goldstein N. IV Complications from tattoos. J Dermatol Surg Oncol. 1979;5:869-78.
59. Jungmann S, Laux P, Bauer TT, et al. From the tattoo studio to the emergency room. Dtsch Arztebl Int. 2016;113:672-5.
60. Lee-Wong M, Karagic M, Silverberg N. Anaphylactic reaction to permanent tattoo ink. Ann Allergy Asthma Immunol. 2009;103:88-9.
61. De Groot AC. Contact allergy to formaldehyde. Br J Dermatol. 2011;164:463.
62. Abiona TC, Balogun JA, Adefuye AS, et al. Body art practices among inmates: Implications for transmission of bloodborne infections. Am J Infect Control. 2010;38:121-9.
63. Jafari S, Copes R, Baharlou S, et al. Tattooing and the risk of transmission of hepatitis C: a systematic review and meta-analysis. Int J Infect Dis. 2010;14:e928-40.
64. Jafari S1, Buxton JA, Afshar K, et al. Tattooing and risk of hepatitis B: a systematic review and meta-analysis. Can J Public Health. 2012;103:207-12.
65. Messahel A, Musgrove B. Infective complications of tattooing and skin piercing. J Infect Pub Health. 2009;2:7-13.
66. Nishioka SA, Gyorkos TW. Tattoos as risk factors for transfusion transmitted diseases. Int J Infect Dis. 2001;5:27-34.
67. Resnick L, Veren K, Salahuddin SZ, et al. Stability and inactivation of HTLV-III/LAV under clinical and laboratory environments. JAMA. 1986;255:1887-91.
68. Doll D. Tattooing in prison and HIV infection. Lancet. 1988;9:66-7.
69. Onder M. Temporary holiday "tattoos" may cause lifelong allergic contact dermatitis when henna is mixed with PPD. J Cosmet Dermatol. 2003;2:126-30.
70. de Groot AC. Side-effects of henna and semi-permanent 'black henna" tattoos: a full review. Contact Dermatitis. 2013;69:1-25.

Chapter 7

Laser Tattoo Removal

Sanjeev J Aurangabadkar

INTRODUCTION

The word tattoo or tattow is derived from a Polynesian word "tatau" as was first described in the 18th century.[1] Tattooing has been in vogue since the ancient times for various reasons such as cultural, religious, and decorative. Single color amateur tattoos are being superseded by complex multicolored decorative tattoos with the current trend being 3D tattoos, optical illusion tattoos, head mandala tattoos and foot tattoos to name a few. Present statistics show that nearly 25% of Australians below 30 years sport at least one tattoo![2] While tattooing has gained popularity, a fair subset of people with tattoos seeks its removal. In the past, before lasers became widely available, limited options existed for tattoo removal. These included dermabrasion, surgical excision, cryotherapy, salabrasion, etc.[3] These methods often led to poor cosmetic results and also scarring in many instances as shown in Figures 7.1 and 7.2. Many a times, individual try many methods to get rid of tattoo leading to complications (Figs. 7.3 and 7.4). The advent of lasers, particularly Q-switched (QS) lasers (and more recently picosecond lasers), has transformed the tattoo removal scenario and lasers have now become the primary treatment modality for tattoo removal.[4]

MECHANISM OF ACTION OF Q-SWITCHED LASERS

Q switching is a method for obtaining energetic pulses from lasers by modulating the intracavity losses—the so-called the Q factor of the laser resonator. The technique is mainly applied for the generation of nanosecond pulses of high energy and peak power with solid-state bulk lasers. These giant pulses are responsible for the unique laser-tissue interaction that is seen with QS lasers.[5] *Q-switched lasers work on the principle of selective photothermolysis*

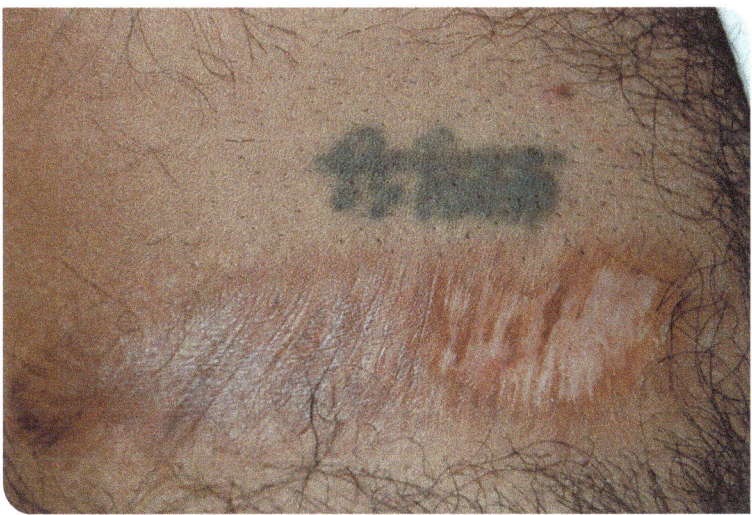

Fig. 7.1: Dermabrasion done for tattoo removal leading to scarring.

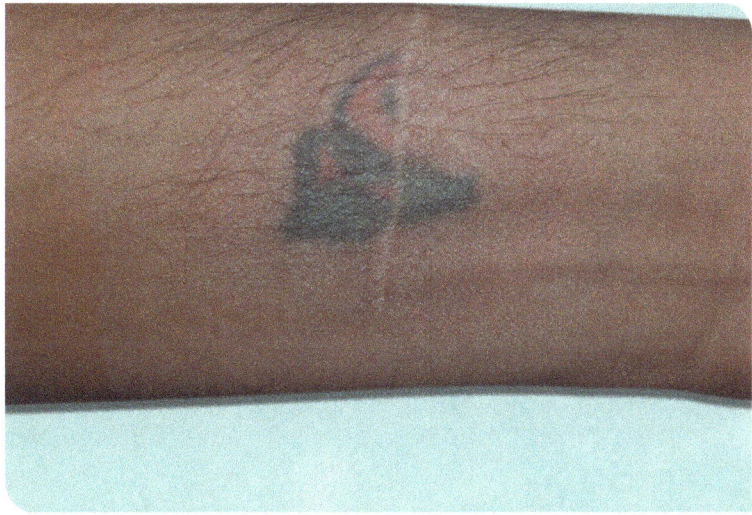

Fig. 7.2: Partial surgical excision of tattoo with ineffective removal and linear scar.

and also produce an additional photoacoustic effect producing shock waves that cause explosion of target.[6] Very high energy, to the tune of 300 mega-watts, is delivered in a very short period of time (5–100 ns) which leads to rapid thermal expansion. This produces shock waves that rupture the targets such as melanosomes and ink particles.[7] The ruptured fragments are cleared by tissue macrophages either to the lymphatic channels or to the regional lymph nodes. Some fragments may be eliminated transepi-dermally. To be selective, the pulse duration of the laser should match the

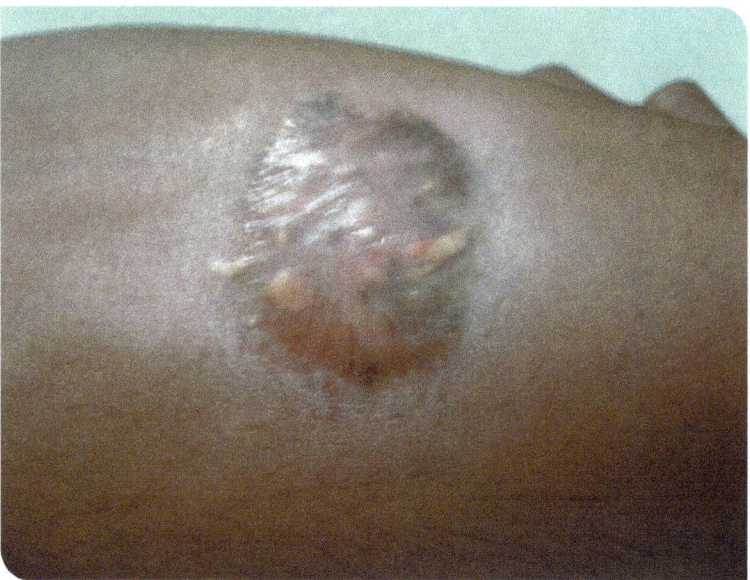

Fig. 7.3: A case of deliberate burns to remove tattoo leading to atrophy with calcinosis cutis.
Source: Dr Shashikumar BM.

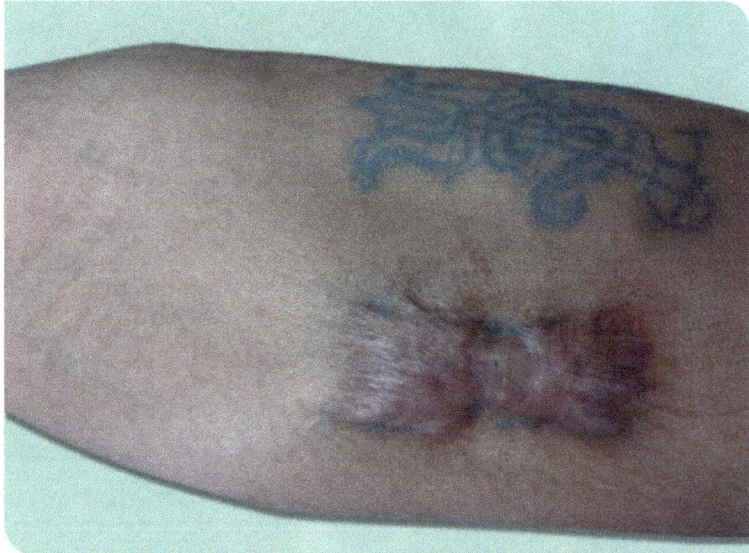

Fig. 7.4: Hypertrophic scar on a tattoo secondary to self-manual dermabrasion.
Source: Dr Shashikumar BM.

thermal relaxation time (TRT) of the target. The estimated TRT of epidermis is 1–10 ms and the TRT of tattoo ink particles is 0.1–10 ns, although some

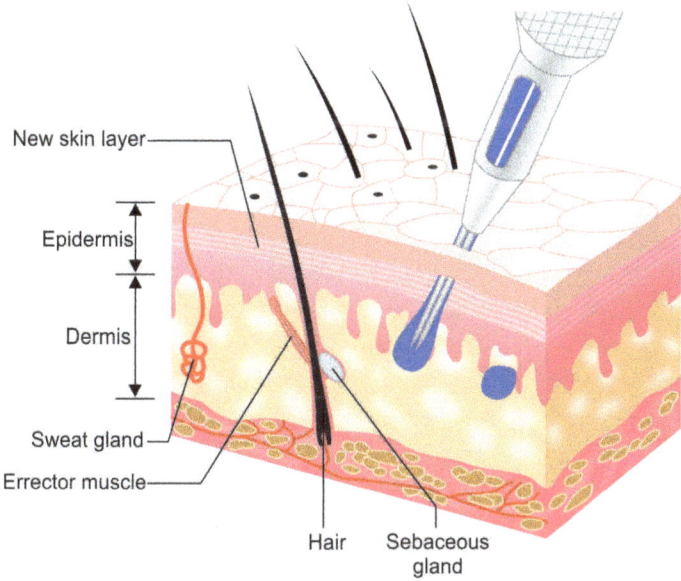

Fig. 7.5: Illustrative diagram showing the depth of placement of tattoo with a tattoo gun.

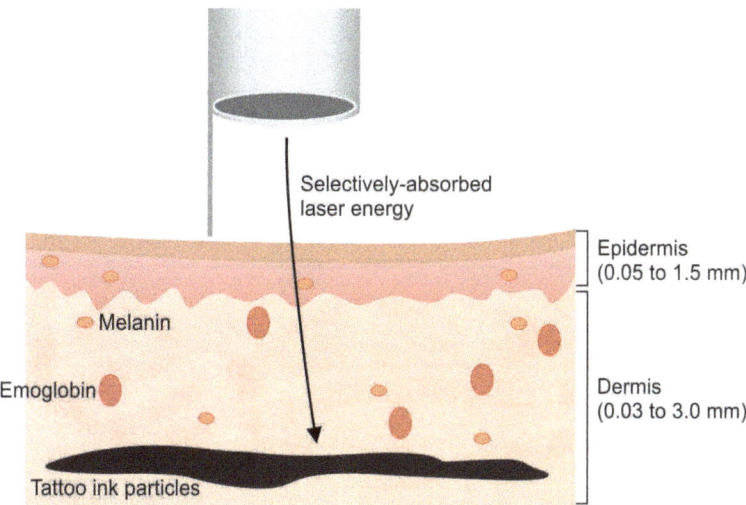

Fig. 7.6: Illustrative diagram showing the selective absorption of laser pulse by tattoo ink in the dermis.

newer estimates are in the range of 10–100 ps. The size of the tattoo ink particles is about 10–100 nm and is generally placed at a depth of 1.1–2.9 mm (Figs. 7.5 and 7.6). Laser tissue interaction produces intracellular steam and vacuole formation, which leads to immediate whitening. An audible popping sound is heard during the procedure due to the photoacoustic effect.[3]

Basic Principles of Q-Switched Lasing

Tattoos consist of thousands of large particles of pigment suspended in the skin.

Q-switched laser delivers energy in an ultra-short duration, typically in nanosecond range with very high peak power. This energy is then selectively absorbed by tattoo ink because of its preferential wavelength and TRT. The surface temperature of the ink particles can rise to thousands of degrees but this energy profile rapidly collapses into a shock wave.[8] This shock wave then propagates throughout the local tissue (the dermis) causing brittle structures (tattoo pigment) to fragment and leads to vibrational damage to cellular structures and rupture of cell membranes.[8] The rapid heating of melanosomes converts cytoplasmic water into steam, which results in intracytoplasmic vacuole formation. Due to this, there is sudden change in light scarring properties of skin, which is evident clinically as whitening or frosting. Frosting prevents further penetration of laser into the skin.[9] The current trends and techniques in laser tattoo removal have attempted to reduce the total number of sessions needed, to shorten the total duration of time required to achieve clearing of tattoos and also to minimize adverse effects. The choice of laser depends on the skin type, tattoo ink, and type of the tattoo to be treated. The characteristics of the laser, i.e. spot size, pulse width, and fluence, are the key to successful treatments. Type of the ink used (organic or inorganic, heavy metals, etc.), amount of ink placed, and the depth of ink placement also affect the outcomes. Until now, multiple sessions spaced over a period of time have been the protocol for tattoo removal. The limitations included incomplete clearance, long total treatment duration, and ineffective removal of some colors. Other problems faced in laser tattoo removal include allergic reactions to certain ink, darkening of cosmetic tattoos, tattoo resistance, etc.

INDICATIONS AND TYPES OF TATTOOS

Amateur Tattoos

They are made of carbon-based ink. They tend to be less dense than professional tattoos. These types of tattoos respond readily to Q-switched laser treatment. Wavelength of 1,064 nm is the preferred wavelength as it targets black ink in the dermis and also can penetrate deep. Generally, less number of sessions is needed for removal as compared to professional tattoos. Figure 7.7 shows a typical black amateur tattoo.

Professional Tattoos

They are more complex and can be multicolored. Inks used include organic (azo dyes) or inorganic compounds (cadmium, mercury, cobalt, copper,

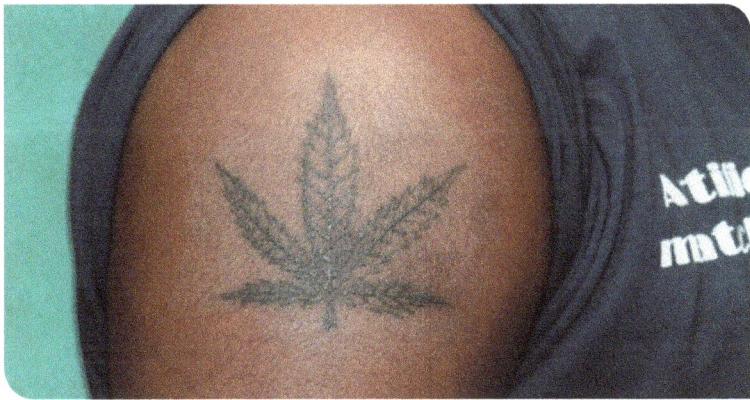

Fig. 7.7: Amateur tattoo on the right arm of a male.

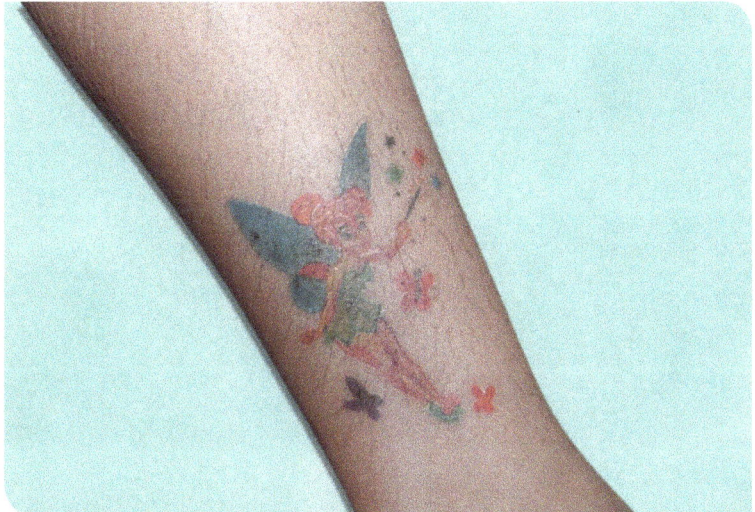

Fig. 7.8: A multicolored professional tattoo.

cinnabar, ferric oxide, TiO_2, carbon ink, etc.).[3] Professional tattoos are more dense and intricate than amateur tattoos. These generally need multiple treatments and yet may not clear fully. Figure 7.8 showcases a typical multicolored professional tattoo on the leg of a female.

The available wavelengths for tattoo removal are shown in Box 7.1.

CONTRAINDICATIONS[10]

The contraindications for performing the lasers on a particular patient should be borne in mind by the clinician all the time. The contraindications can be relative or absolute are listed hereunder.

Box 7.1: Wavelengths for tattoo removal.

- Wavelengths used for tattoo removal:
- Q-switched Nd:YAG 1,064 nm—blue black tattoos
- Q-switched Nd:YAG 532 nm—red tattoo ink
- Q-switched 755 nm alex—purple and teal colors
- Q-switched ruby 694 nm—green color
- Picosecond 755 nm alex—blue and green color tattoos
- Q-switched 660 nm—green color
- Q-switched 585 nm—sky blue color

Absolute Contraindications

- Associated photoaggravated skin diseases and medical illness, for example, systemic lupus erythematosus.
- Treatment area with active cutaneous infections, for example, herpes labialis, staphylococcal infections.
- Unstable vitiligo and psoriasis for risk of koebnerization of treated area
- Tattoo granuloma.
- Localized allergic reactions can occur with almost any color ink and result in urticaria and granulomatous reactions. If a patient exhibits a cutaneous reaction within a tattoo, QS laser treatment should be used with caution. After QS laser treatment, the ink particles are mobilized, potentially triggering an allergic response. Rarely systemic allergic reactions may occur, particularly common in patients exhibiting a localized allergic response.

Relative Contraindications

In the following situations, laser has to be used cautiously, and, after proper counseling of the patient; use of laser in these situations depends on individual situation and on treating physician's judgment.

- Keloid and keloidal tendencies
- Patient on isotretinoin. (A large multicenter study in India has shown QS laser treatment is safe in such patients but caution has to be exercised and patients carefully followed up.)
- History of herpes simplex or history of herpes for increased risk of reactivation: This risk should be seriously considered prior to performing the procedure. If the treating physician decides to perform the procedure, the risk and benefit should be explained to the patient and the procedure should be performed after proper informed consent and only after a course of acyclovir.

- Patient who is not cooperative or has unrealistic expectations:
  - Pregnancy or nursing
  - Body dysmorphic disorder
  - Photosensitizing medication such as tetracyclines, thiazides
  - Gold therapy (used for the treatment of arthritis)
  - Livedo reticularis (can be exacerbated with heat exposure by laser)
  - Erythema ab igne
  - Seizure disorder
  - Melanoma or suspected melanoma in the treatment area.

PATIENT SELECTION AND COUNSELING[11,12]

Patient selection needs utmost care on the part of the clinician.
- A general medical history, current medical conditions and medications, allergies, past surgeries, including bleeding tendencies and wound healing (response of previous skin injuries whether they heal with hyperpigmentation or hypopigmentation, response to previous laser sessions if any taken) should be obtained.
- Thorough counseling of the patient and an informed written consent completes the baseline step required for initiating therapy.
- Good pretreatment photographs are mandatory, as in any esthetic procedure. Scarring often occurs during tattoo placement and may be unmasked and become more noticeable once the ink is removed. Serial photographs should therefore be taken at successive visits. Ideally the photographs should be taken with same or similar camera equipment and settings, distance, uniform light and background.

PREOPERATIVE PREPARATION

Sun Protection

Epidermal melanin produced by ultraviolet (UV) light exposure may interfere with laser treatment and increase the risks for scarring, hypopigmentation or hyperpigmentation. It is very important to ensure that the patient is not tanned.[13-15] To check for tanning, it is wise to compare the color of the potential treatment site to that of an unexposed skin site, similar to the buttock or axilla. If a tan is present, treatment should be delayed until the tan has faded as much as possible in the treatment area. Use of broad-spectrum sun protection creams with UVA coverage is crucial. Protective clothing and bleaching creams can be useful in treating the tan. Patients with darker skin types and tanned patients are advised to apply hydroquinone-containing compounds (2–4%) or other lightening agents preoperatively to minimize the risk of postinflammatory hyperpigmentation (PIH).

Oral Retinoids

It has been recommended that patients on oral retinoid therapy should not undergo laser treatment of pigmented lesions and tattoos for 6–12 months following discontinuation of the medication, as they have an increased risk of keloidal scar formation.[3] Proper evidence to support such a recommendation in Indian patients, particularly for epidermal lesions, is lacking. However, caution is advised while treating all patients with history of recent administration of isotretinoin.

Eye Protection

The QS laser light can cause permanent retinal damage and vision loss.[16] Precautions include protective clothing, goggles, masks and laser cone containment devices which should be used with every patient. Eye protection in the form of optically coated glasses or goggles for the specific laser being used is necessary. All persons present in the room during laser treatment must also wear appropriate eye protection. The eye wear should block the wavelength being used and the lens should provide an optical density (OD) for at least four. Laser protective eye shields (anodized external metal eyecup) must be used when treating periorbital lesions. When treating eyelids, a metal corneal eye shield should be placed on the eye using topical anesthesia to protect the globe.

Test Patch

A test patch helps to determine the treatment parameters for an individual. It is also helpful in medicolegal situations. In particular, it is advisable for all beginning practitioners to perform laser test spots in all patients prior to treating an entire lesion, since skin type and color do not always perfectly predict the response to treatment. Even seasoned experts may need to perform small test spots, particularly where response to treatment cannot be judged properly. Always evaluate the patient 4–8 weeks after the test spots.[3,12,14]

Box 7.2 shows the check list before performing laser surgery.

Anesthesia

The Q-switched laser treatment usually does not require anesthesia. However, if a large area needs to be treated, topical eutectic mixture of local anesthetic (EMLA) should be applied under occlusion 1–2 hours before the procedure.[17,18]

Laser Procedure

Selecting the appropriate laser parameters is of paramount importance while executing the treatment.

Fluence

It is always preferable to begin with the lowest energy fluence that produces a visible response. Fluence may be increased if response is suboptimal. If epidermal debris is significant, the fluence should be lowered.[19]

Spot Size

For dermal lesions and tattoos, the spot size that elicits immediate brisk whitening on laser irradiation should be selected. Larger spot sizes allow deeper penetration and produce less tissue splatter.[20] The exact spot size selection will depend on the laser system being used, the type and size of the tattoo and the wavelength being used.

Endpoint of Treatment

- Appropriate endpoints are essential to ensure optimum outcome. With the QS laser, the endpoint of treatment is immediate whitening of the lesion. Higher fluences may produce pinpoint bleeding and blistering.
- *Repetition rate*: Choose higher frequency, i.e. 5–10 Hz while doing large area. For smaller discrete lesions a frequency of 2–3 Hz gives better control.

  Figures 7.9 and 7.10 show an amateur tattoo before treatment. Figures 7.11 and 7.12 show immediate whitening of the treated area.

Laser Technique

After choosing the correct spot size and the energy fluence (J/cm^2), laser treatment is performed with the handpiece held perpendicular to the lesion and the entire area is covered with minimal overlap (up to 10%). QS laser

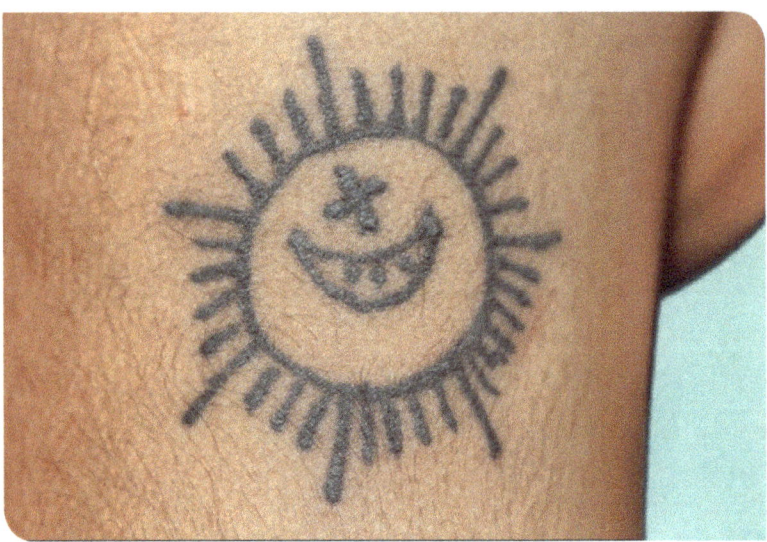

Fig. 7.9: Amateur tattoo before treatment.

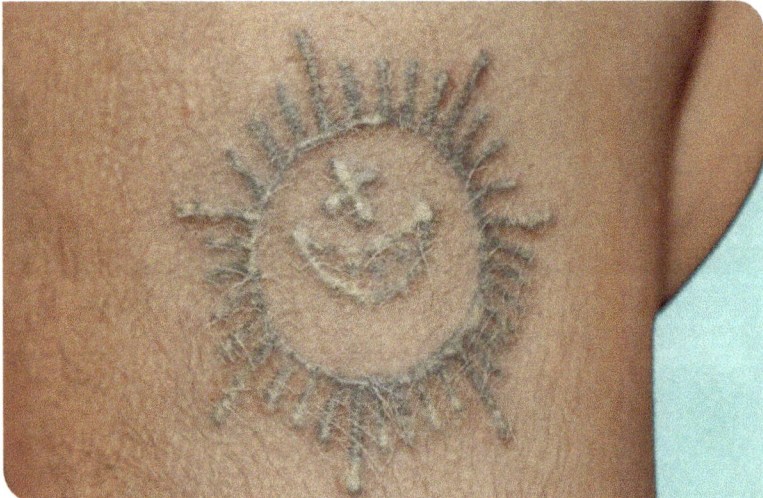

Fig. 7.10: Immediate post-treatment view showing whitening of the lesion.

treatment will produce an immediate whitening of the lesion. Pinpoint bleeding may occur if very high fluences are used. The entire lesion is covered in one pass. A popping sound is heard with each laser shot as the cells containing melanin or ink particles explode. Laser pulses are placed close to each other with minimum overlap. The area is cooled with ice packs or air cooling (e.g. Zimmer) just before and after laser pulses to avoid a buildup of heat and to prevent collateral tissue damage.

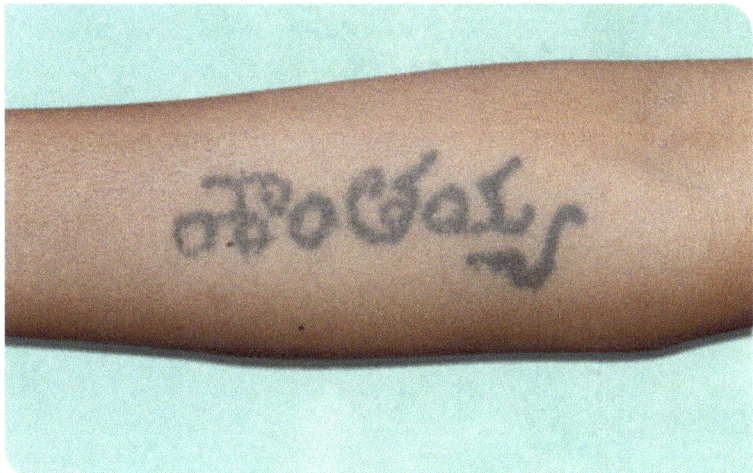

Fig. 7.11: Amateur tattoo on the forearm.

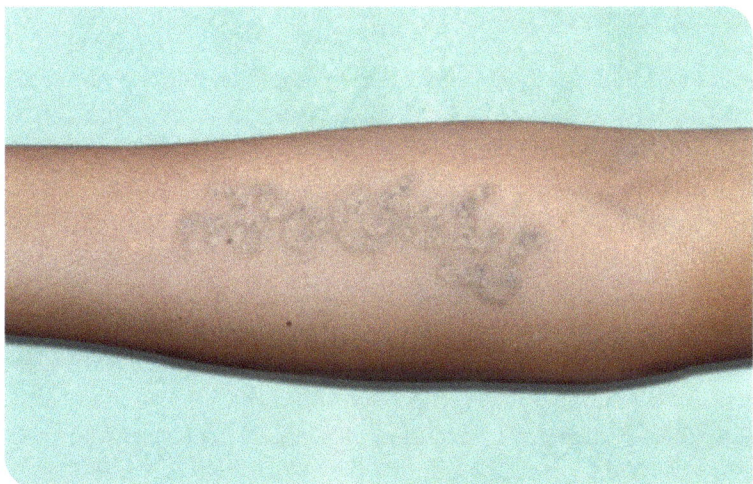

Fig. 7.12: Amateur tattoo on the forearm immediately after Q-switched neodymium: yttrium-aluminum-garnet showing brisk whitening.

Number of Sessions

Tattoos may need 2–20 sessions for successful lightening. Professional tattoos require more treatment sessions for eradication. Amateur tattoos are less dense and are often made up of carbon-based ink that responds more readily to QS laser treatment. Traumatic tattoos are more superficial with minimal pigment and clear with one or two treatments. Gunpowder and firework tattoos need more care while treating as the implanted material has the potential to ignite and result in pox-like scars after treatment.

Table 7.1: Factors affecting number of treatments needed for tattoo removal.		
Characteristics	*Less sessions*	*More sessions*
Tattoo type	Amateur, traumatic	Professional, cosmetic
Color	Black	Multicolored
Age	Old	New
Intensity	Faded	Dark
Layering	No	Yes
Skin type	Fairer	Darker
Scarring	No	Yes
Location	Proximal	Distal

Table 7.1 highlights the factors affecting the number of treatments needed for tattoo removal.

Interval between Sessions

Treatment should be done at least 6–8 weeks apart. While treating tattoos longer intervals are advisable. Continued clearance of the lesion occurs due to removal of pigment by macrophages and lymphatics between treatments. Optimal interval between treatments therefore needs to be determined on an individual basis.[20]

Q-Switched lasers are very effective for dark-blue, black and green tattoos, whereas red and yellow tattoos are more difficult to treat as the absorption spectrum for these colors lies in the 500–600 nm spectrum (green light). The Q-switched neodymium:yttrium-aluminum-garnet (QS Nd:YAG) laser has a 532 nm wavelength that can be used for red ink but use of high fluence is difficult in Indian patients due to the darker skin types. The QS 660 nm wavelength can also be used for yellow or red colors. The risk of dyschromias is high with these wavelengths. Pigments which contain iron oxide tend to darken on exposure to laser; hence a test patch is desirable. While amateur tattoos can be removed in fewer sessions, professional tattoos which are intricate and multicolored may need more sessions. Some professional tattoos may not clear completely, in spite of repeated treatments, and a ghost image of the design may be left behind.[21-28]

Figures 7.13 and 7.14 show an amateur tattoo on the arm of a young female before and after four 1,064 nm QS Nd:YAG laser sessions. Figures 7.15 and 7.16 show amateur tattoos on the chin before and after 1,064 nm QS Nd:YAG laser treatment.

Figures 7.17 to 7.20 show amateur tattoos before and after QS Nd:YAG laser demonstrating the excellent response to therapy.

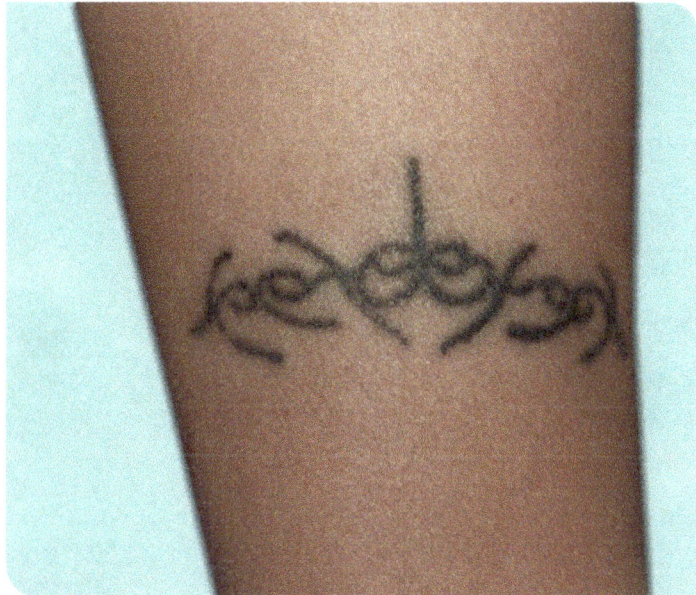

Fig. 7.13: Amateur tattoo on the arm.

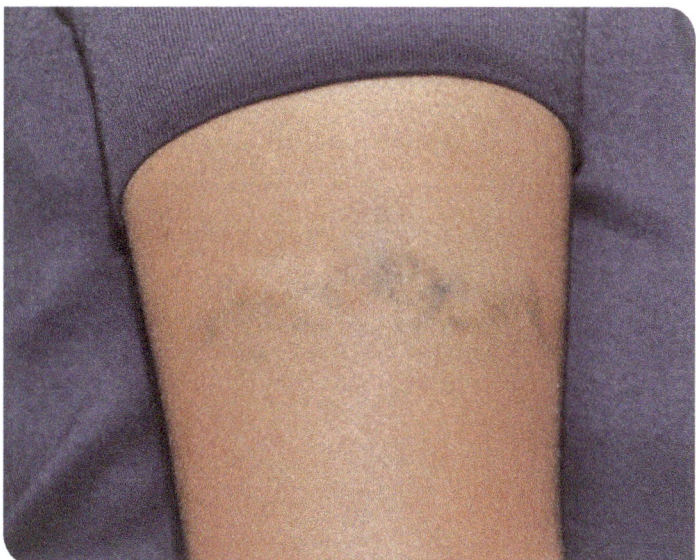

Fig. 7.14: Amateur tattoo on the arm after four 1,064 nm QS Nd:YAG laser sessions.

TRAUMATIC TATTOOS

These tattoos occur after road traffic accidents where asphalt granules may be deposited in the skin. Usually, a small amount of pigment as deposited

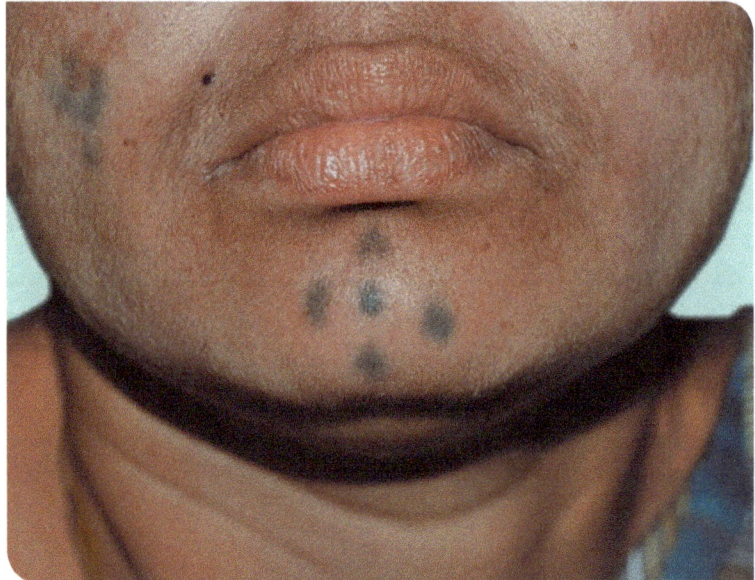

Fig. 7.15: Amateur tattoos on chin.

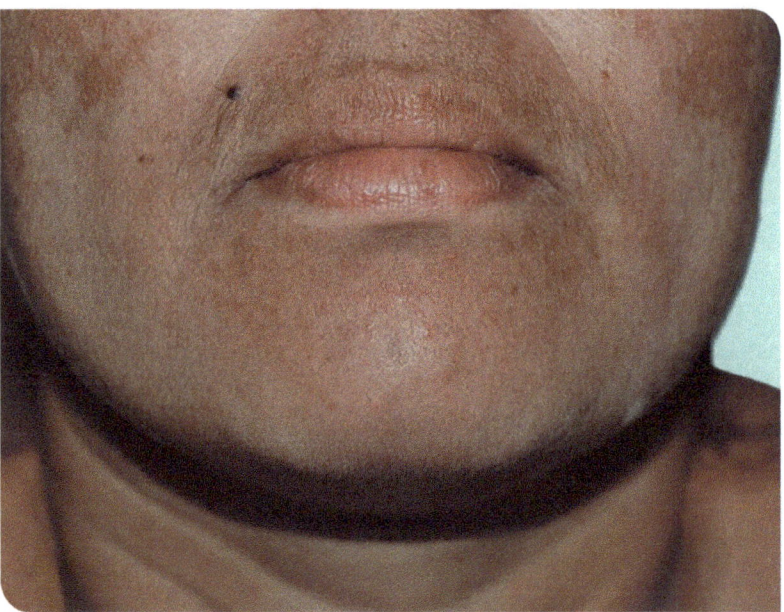

Fig. 7.16: Amateur tattoos on chin after a single 1,064 nm QS Nd:YAG laser treatment.

superficially in the skin and often clears with one or two treatments with 1,064 nm Q-switched Nd:YAG laser.[28,29]

Figure 7.21 shows a traumatic tattoo on the forehead.

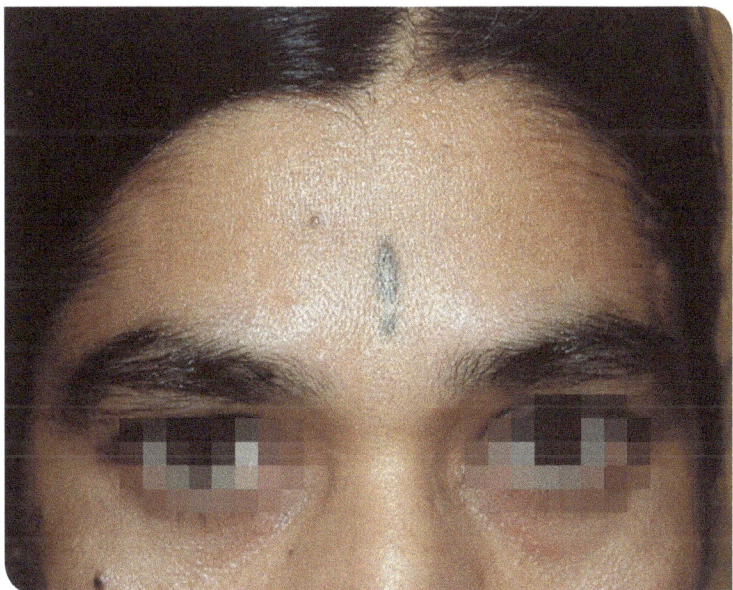

Fig. 7.17: Amateur tattoo on forehead.

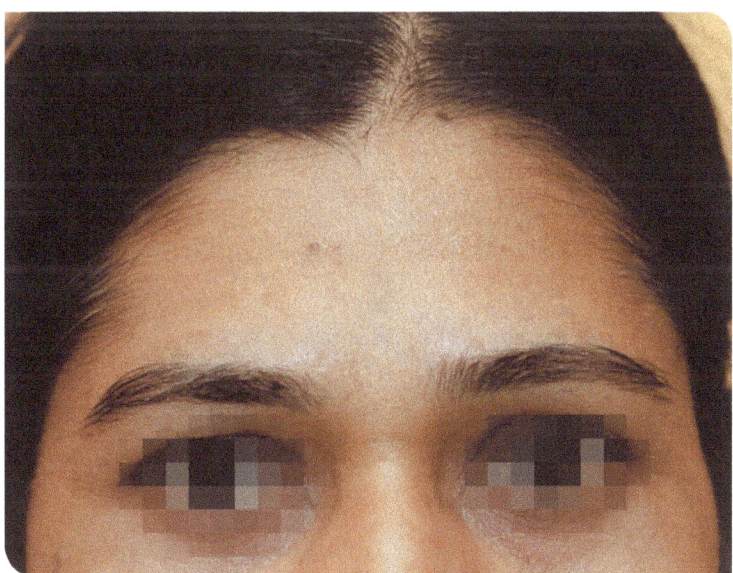

Fig. 7.18: Amateur tattoo after six QS Nd:YAG laser sessions.

COSMETIC TATTOOS

These tattoos are usually red, white or flesh colored. The pigment is placed to create areolae after breast reconstruction surgery or is in the form of lip

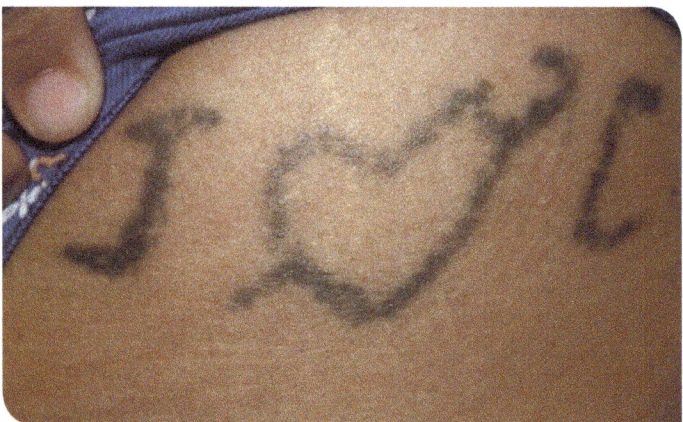

Fig. 7.19: A faded old amateur tattoo on the hip.

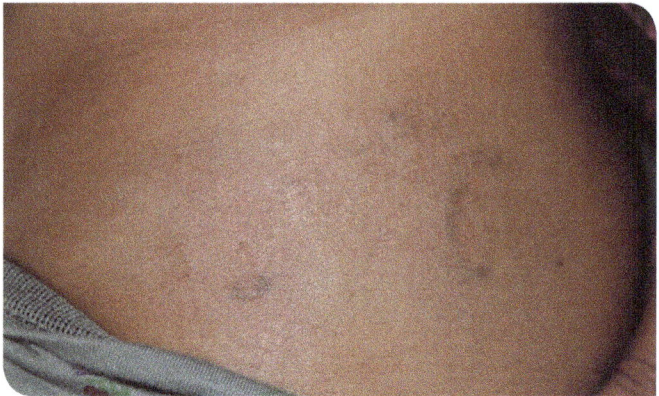

Fig. 7.20: Excellent response to QS Nd:YAG laser after five sessions.

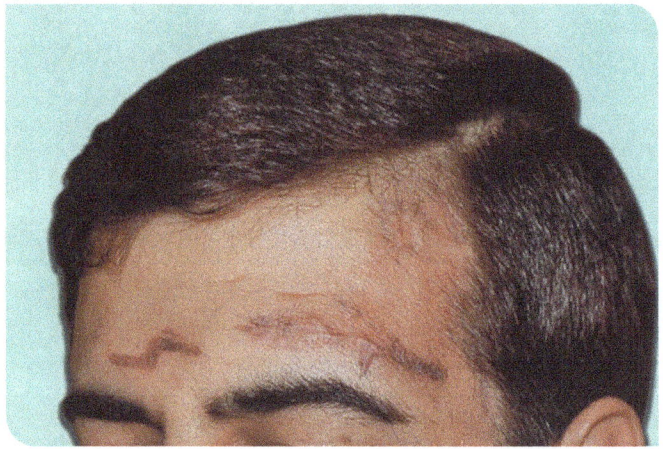

Fig. 7.21: Traumatic tattoo on the forehead after road traffic accident.

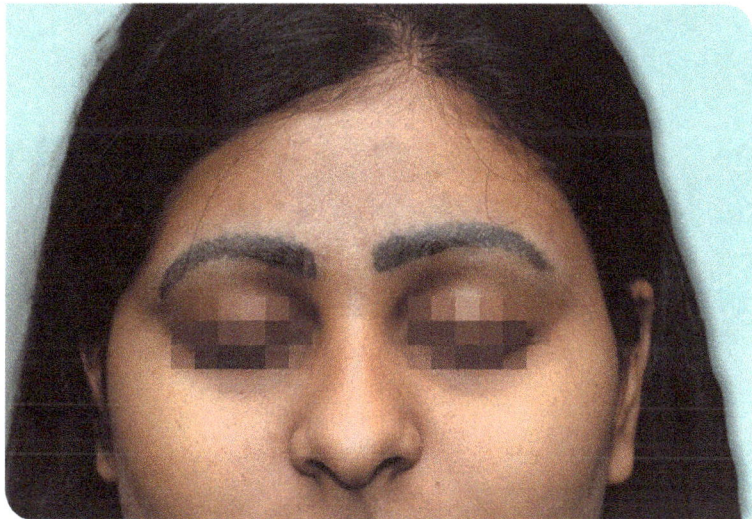

Fig. 7.22: Cosmetic tattoo—permanent make up of eye brows.

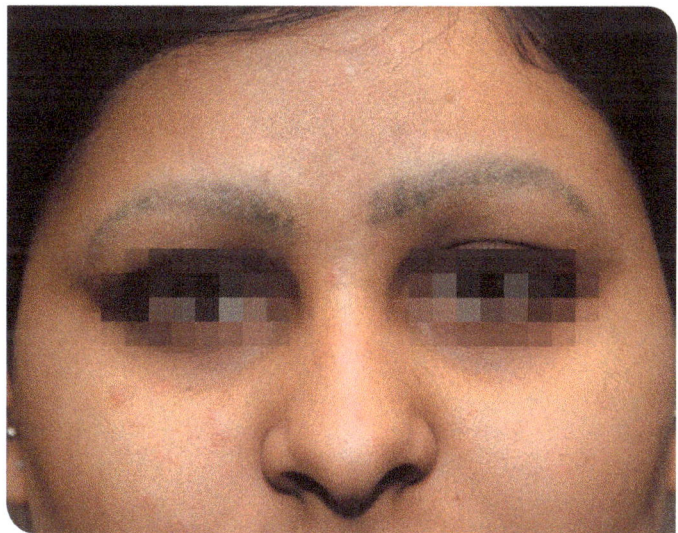

Fig. 7.23: After four sessions of QS Nd:YAG laser treatment.

liner tattoos. Pigment darkening may occur after laser therapy of these tattoos, hence, test patches are recommended. The patients should follow-up for 6–8 weeks after a test patch. If there is no darkening of the test patch and the tattoo lightens or fades, treatment can be undertaken for the rest of the tattoo. However, if the tattoo darkens, it is best to avoid further treatments.[30,31] Figures 7.22 and 7.23 show a case of cosmetic tattoo (permanent eyebrows) before and after QS Nd:YAG laser treatment.

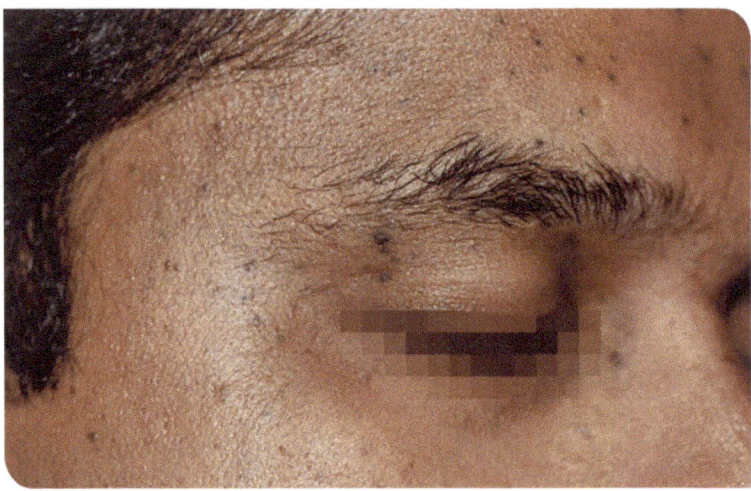

Fig. 7.24: Firework tattoos on the right side of face and eyelid after a fire cracker injury.

GUNPOWDER AND FIREWORK TATTOOS

Care should be taken while treating these types of tattoos, as the implanted material has the potential to ignite, and pox-like scars can develop. A test spot is mandatory in such cases and only after evaluating the patient after 6–8 weeks should further treatments be taken up.[32,33]

Figure 7.24 shows multiple hyperpigmented scattered spots of firework tattoos on the right side of face and eyelid in a male patient.

The Kirby-Desai Scale has been proposed to be used to estimate the approximate number of sessions needed for a given tattoo based on the following factors:[34]

- Fitzpatrick skin type
- Location
- Color
- Amount of ink used
- Scarring and tissue damage
- Ink layering.

Each of these six factors is given numerical score and the total of these will give an estimate of the approximate number of sessions required for tattoo removal.

NEWER TECHNIQUES FOR LASER TATTOO REMOVAL

The limitations of conventional protocol of tattoo removal led to the development of newer techniques.[4] These limitations include a long total duration of treatment (interval of 6–8 weeks between treatments), ink retention despite multiple sessions (which could be due to wrong or ineffective wavelength choice for multicolored tattoos, poor technique, insufficient interval between sessions, etc.), ghosting (shadow or outline of the residual tattoo), and complications such as hyper- and hypopigmentation, blistering and scarring. The newer protocols attempt to overcome these short comings by modifying the technique or combining multiple lasers to achieve optimal results and minimize adverse effects.

The newer techniques for laser tattoo removal are:
- R20 technique
- R0 technique
- Combining fractional lasers with Q-switched lasers.

R20 Method

Tattoo removal in a single laser session, based on method of repeated exposure.[35,36] Four treatment passes are done with an interval of 20 minutes between passes. Immediate whitening is seen on the first pass with little or no whitening on subsequent passes. Kossida et al. in a study found that treatment with the R20 method was much more effective than conventional single-pass laser treatment.[35]

After removing the EMLA cream and cleaning the area, first pass with the QS Nd:YAG laser at 1,064 nm wavelength is made. There is immediate whitening of the treated area. This is due to the intracellular steam formation and gas bubble formation. Upon waiting for 20 minutes following the first pass, the gas bubbles are cleared due to absorption of the gases whereby the next laser pass can be delivered. This allows further bombardment of the tattoo particles by the QS Nd:YAG laser pulses. Energy is either constant as the first pass of lowered by 10–20%. A total of four such passes are made. The tattoo clears well after this over time. Based on the response another R20 session can be done after an interval of 6–8 weeks. The drawback of R20 is the long waiting time in the clinic for the patient and the physician. The patient will need to be there for over 2 hours. This is a limitation of this technique. It also can require multiple R20 sessions to eliminate the ink completely, which still may not be possible. Although reported safe in type 1–4 skin, in pigmented skin the overall incidence of blistering, scarring, and pigmentary alteration can be more (Fig. 7.25).

R0 Method

Repeated exposure on same day without waiting period can be performed by applying perfluorodecalin (a perfluorocarbon compound, commercially available as "Zero-W") immediately after lasing (Fig. 7.26).[37] This compound

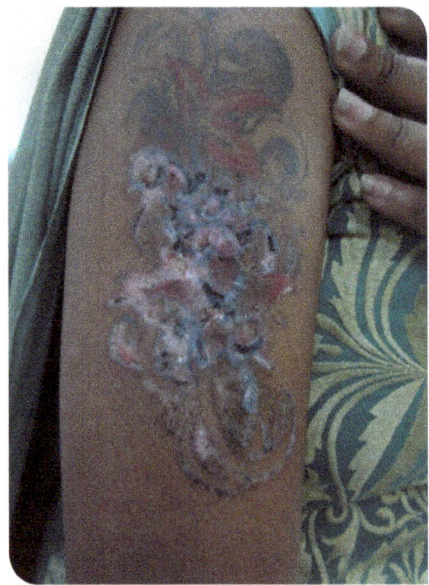

Fig. 7.25: Severe burns secondary R20 method of laser tattoo removal. *Source*: Dr Shashikumar BM.

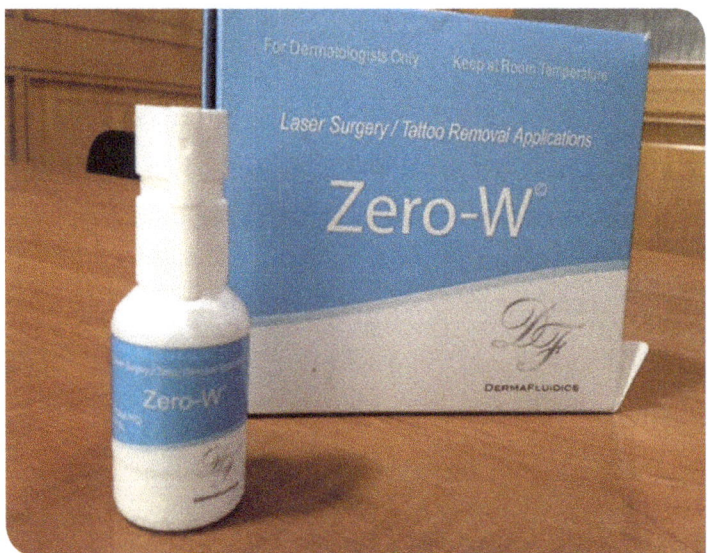

Fig. 7.26: Perfluorodecalin spray available commercially as Zero-W.

dissolves the gas bubbles formed upon initial laser exposure thus opening the optical window by reducing scatter. This allows an immediate next pass to be performed without the waiting time of 20 minutes as in the R20 technique.

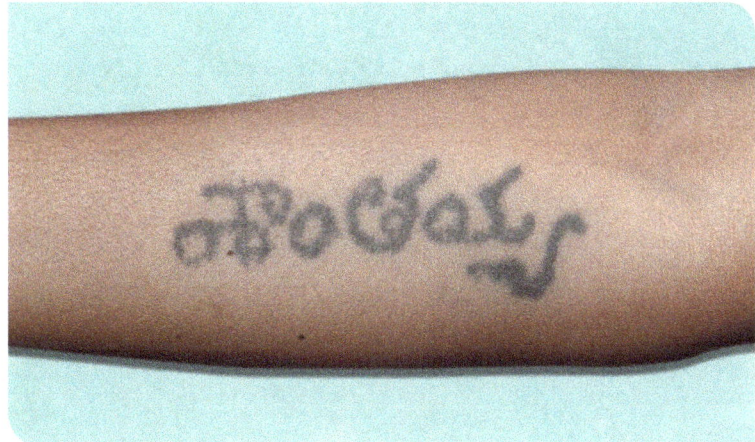

Fig. 7.27: Amateur tattoo on the forearm.

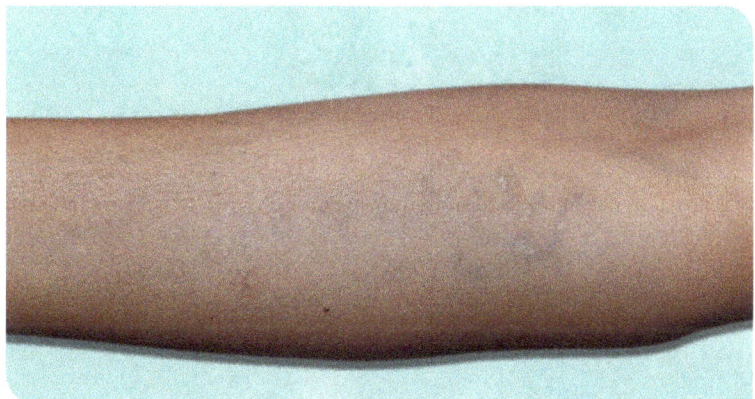

Fig. 7.28: Amateur tattoo after a single "R0" session with QS Nd:YAG.

This method significantly cuts down on the waiting time for the patient in the clinic unlike the R20 method. The only downside is the additional cost of the perfluorodecalin and its availability.

Results are similar to R20 and overall both these techniques score over the standard tattoo removal methods by reducing the length of time taken for fading of the tattoo.

Some examples of improvement with the R0 method can be seen in Figures 7.27 to 7.32.

Combining Lasers

Monotherapy with Q-switched laser is often effective for tattoo removal but combining Q-switched laser with an ablative or nonablative laser may

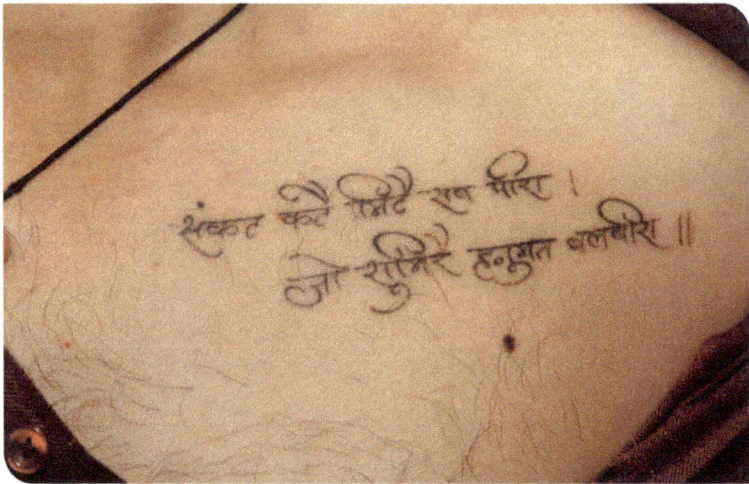

Fig. 7.29: A fresh tattoo on the chest with well-defined margins and dark color.

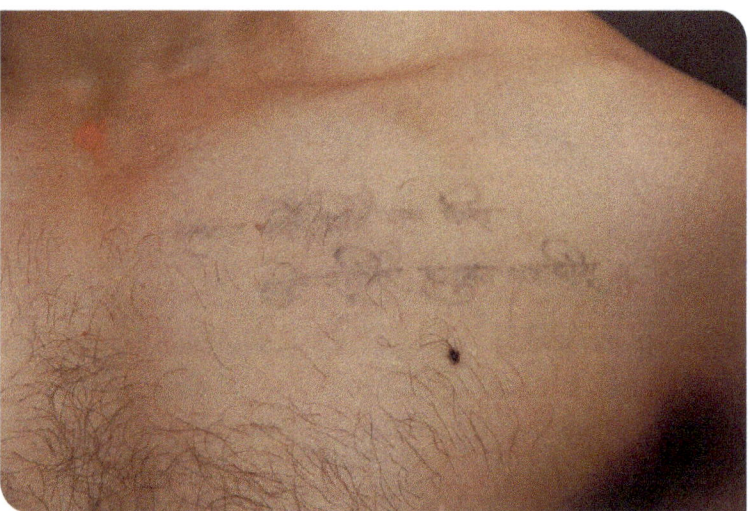

Fig. 7.30: After two "R0" sessions with QS Nd:YAG laser, excellent clearing of the pigment.

yield faster clearing, minimize number of sessions and reduce side effects. Combination can be in any order.

Ablative fractional laser followed by Q-switched laser helps to reduce blister formation. A study by Weiss and Geronimus found that after multiple sessions of Q-switched laser followed immediately by either nonablative fractional resurfacing (NAFR) or ablative fractional resurfacing (AFR) increases tattoo clearance, eliminates blistering, shortens recovery and diminishes treatment induced hypopigmentation. They noted the addition

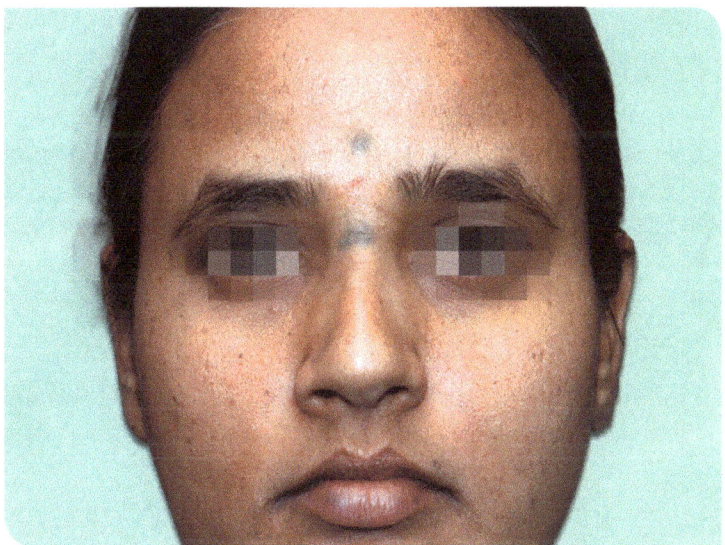

Fig. 7.31: Amateur tattoo on the nose and glabella.

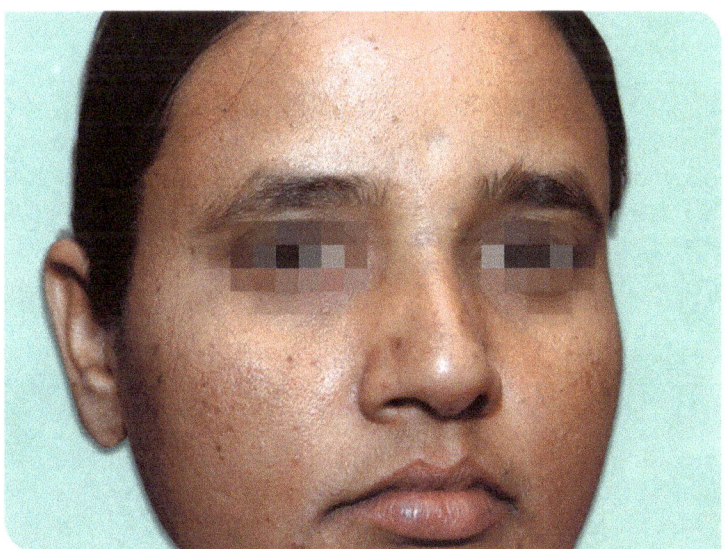

Fig. 7.32: After single "R0" session with three passes. Note the mild depressed scarring which was unmasked after tattoo removal.

of AFR to Q-switched laser enhances the rate of pigment clearance. Addition of NAFR to Q-switched laser may decrease the degree of treatment-induced hypopigmentation.[38]

Marini et al. proposed a combination of fractional Er:YAG (erbium-doped yttrium aluminum garnet) laser skin conditioning followed by Q-switched

Nd:YAG laser for laser tattoo removal. In their two step technique, they used a fractional Er:YAG laser to drill micro holes into the skin which was followed by Q-switched laser treatment. According to the authors, this fractional Er:YAG laser conditioning protects the skin from damages at higher fluences by allowing the escape of gases through these micro holes and thus relieving the internal pressure generated by Q-switched laser treatment. This also aided in repeating the next pass after 20 minutes. They concluded that this procedure led to a 30% reduction in the number of sessions.[39]

Factors affecting tattoo removal: Bencini et al. studied the variables influencing the outcomes in Q-switched laser tattoo removal. The authors assessed the prognostic factors affecting the outcomes in a large cohort of patients and found that smoking, the presence of colors other than black and red, a tattoo larger than 30 cm^2, a tattoo located on the feet or legs or older than 36 months, high color density, treatment intervals of 8 weeks or less, and development of a darkening phenomenon were associated with a reduced clinical response to treatment.[40]

Picosecond Lasers

Current Q-switched laser has pulse duration in nanosecond (10^{-9} of a second). If the pulse duration is narrowed further, the peak energy of the laser beam becomes very high. The picosecond lasers have a pulse duration of 10^{-12} of a second. This results in more rapid heating of the tattoos and finer fragmentation.[41] The lymphatic elimination of these finer particles is easier resulting in faster clearing of the tattoos. The picosecond lasers with pulse durations in the range of 450–750 ps were introduced commercially in the early part of 2013. At present, there are three or more systems with a wavelength of 755 nm and 1,064 nm and pulse duration of 450–750 ps.

Au et al. analyzed the incidence of bulla formation after tattoo treatment using the combination of the picoseconds alexandrite laser and a fractionated carbon dioxide (CO_2) laser ablation.[42] In their study, 32% of patients treated with the picoseconds laser alone experienced blistering, whereas none of the patients treated with the combination developed blistering. The study showed a statistically significant decrease in bulla formation associated with tattoo treatment when fractionated CO_2 ablation was added to the picosecond alexandrite laser.[15]

Because of the shorter wavelength of the alexandrite and the thermal effects of the fractional CO_2 the risk for hyper- and hypopigmentation is high, caution needs to be exercised while treating dark skin.

Recent studies by Brauer et al. demonstrated the efficacy of 755 nm picosecond laser in treating blue and green tattoos.[43] They demonstrated 75% clearance in just 1 or 2 treatment. Saedi et al. also reported similar efficacy. However, they also reported complications such as hypo- and hyperpigmentation at 3 months follow-up in few of their patients.[44] Although effective and safe in white skin, their safety remains to be evaluated in pigmented skin. Furthermore, the cost of these machines is currently very high. Hence they are not yet widely available.

Combination of Imiquimod and Q-switched Laser

Imiquimod is a topical immune response modulator. Topical application of imiquimod alone is known to fade the tattoos to some extent when applied immediately after tattooing. Based on this finding, it was postulated that imiquimod interferes with tattoo pigment phagocytosis and prevents tattoo maturation. Application of laser recreates the biological scene similar to early tattoos. Wherein most of the tattoo pigmented lies freely in the tissue. Thus, it was postulated that combining imiquimod with a laser could increase the efficacy of both modalities.

Elsaie et al. evaluated imiquimod and Q-switched YAG laser (QSYL) in the treatment of tattoos and reported more favorable outcome in the tattoos treatment with combination than tattoos treated alone or with placebo.[45] However, Ricotti et al. studied 20 patients with daily application of imiquimod cream and 4–6 weekly application of QSYL for five sessions and reported imiquimod as ineffective combination. Furthermore they also reported more complications on imiquimod treated site.[46] Based on the limited studies, the use of imiquimod in combination with Q-switched laser remains controversial as of now.

Diascopy in Combination with QSYL

Murphy reported a simple and novel technique to reduce the pain and decrease epidermal damage during laser tattoo removal.[47] The technique consists of application of a glass microscope slide firmly on the treatment area. This applied pressure results in evacuating the blood from capillary plexus. The laser pulse is then applied through the glass slide.

In a study of 31 patients, he reported significantly less pain and less epidermal damage with this technique.

Dermal Scatter Reduction

Light scattering properties of skin and hemoglobin prevent effective penetration of the laser into the skin, which ultimately reduces its clinical efficacy in clearance of deeper tattoos. This becomes more problematic when one tries to remove the colored tattoos since shorter wavelengths (532 nm and 755 nm) are used to treat them. These shorter wavelengths have limited penetration depth.

If an optical clearing agent, such as glycerol, dimethyl sulfoxide, and glucose, is applied to the skin before laser irradiation; because of its high refractive index, hyperosmosis, and biocompatibility into skin, these agents reduce skin scattering of laser beam. This not only allows deeper penetration but also delivery of higher effective energies.

Fox and Diven did the first human study using this concept. They applied glycerol after removing stratum corneum using the low-pressure transdermal delivery device and reported increased efficiency of laser tattoo removal.[48]

Microencapsulation of Tattoo Ink

In recent years, scientists have designed permanent but easily removable ink using a combination of organic and inorganic inks (e.g. β-carotene and iron oxide). This pigment is then stabilized by a transparent microencapsulation technique using polymethylmethacrylate beads.[8] The pigment in this microsphere can easily be targeted using a pigment specific wavelength. This will result in breakage of microspheres and exposing the ink to the body's defense mechanism. In an unpublished data Klitzman et al. demonstrated 80% clearance of tattoo in a single session using microencapsulated tattoo ink in guinea pig and hairless rats.[14] Although promising modality for faster tattoo removal, there are no published data in humans and its safety and efficacy needs further evaluation. Recently one such brand is available in United States as the Infinitink˙ (Freedom Ink, USA).[49]

POSTOPERATIVE INSTRUCTIONS[20]

- Broad-spectrum sunscreens with good UVA/UVB coverage are recommended before and throughout the treatment period.
- Immediately after laser treatment, the treated area appears abraded, and inflamed. Apply ice packs till burning sensation subsides, then apply a layer of antibiotic such as mupirocin and cover with gauze. Patient is instructed to clean the area with copious amount of water and apply the ointment twice daily till lesions heal. Healing can take around 5–10 days.
- Oral antibiotics may be used, if considered essential, but are not mandatory. Anti-inflammatory agents may be needed while treating large lesions. Patient should be instructed to avoid sun exposure and cosmetics on the treated area. Treatments are scheduled at an interval of 6–8 weeks.
- Patients are instructed to apply an antibiotic ointment or petrolatum ointment for about a week after procedure. Strict sun protection is advised for darker patients. Ice packs may be used after the procedure to minimize discomfort.
- Postprocedure bleaching agents may be used but only after the crust subsides.

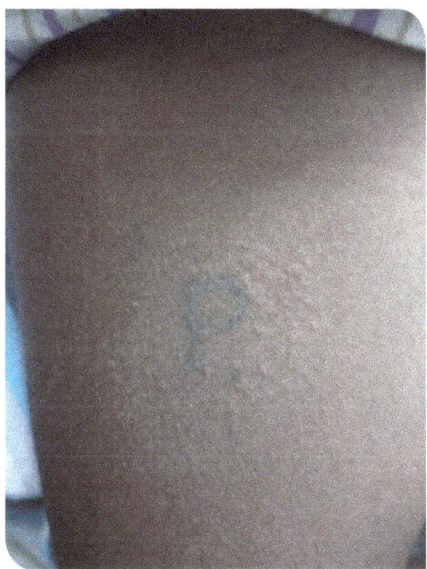

Fig. 7.33: Allergic rash to topical eutectic mixture of local anesthetic. *Source*: Dr Shashikumar BM.

COMPLICATIONS AND THEIR MANAGEMENT[20]

Complications are encountered more frequently in darker skin type which may be minor and transient or major and persistent. The risk of complications increases with more aggressive treatments, poor priming, multiple treatments and choosing inappropriate laser systems and in unrealistic patients. Some of the complications which demand considerations are:

- Allergic to topical anesthetic agent (Fig. 7.33)
- Thermal burns—pain, petechiae, purpura (Fig. 7.34), blister formation (Figs. 7.35 and 7.36)
- Postinflammatory hyperpigmentation resolves with time; some patients may need bleaching agents such as hydroquinone along with sunscreens.
- Postinflammatory hypopigmentation (Fig. 7.37) may persist for several weeks to months and may be difficult to treat. Phototherapy may be used to treat the hypopigmentation. Topical immunomodulators such as pimecrolimus and tacrolimus may be tried in these cases. Targeted phototherapy with 308–311 nm UVB excimer light can also be tried, once weekly till improvement is noted. An average of 15–20 sessions is needed to see a good response. If no improvement is seen in 15 odd sessions then it can be considered as treatment failure.
- Textural changes and scarring (Fig. 7.38)
- Darkening of tattoo pigment, especially flesh colored cosmetic tattoos. Red tattoos can turn black, if it occurs, it is difficult to treat.

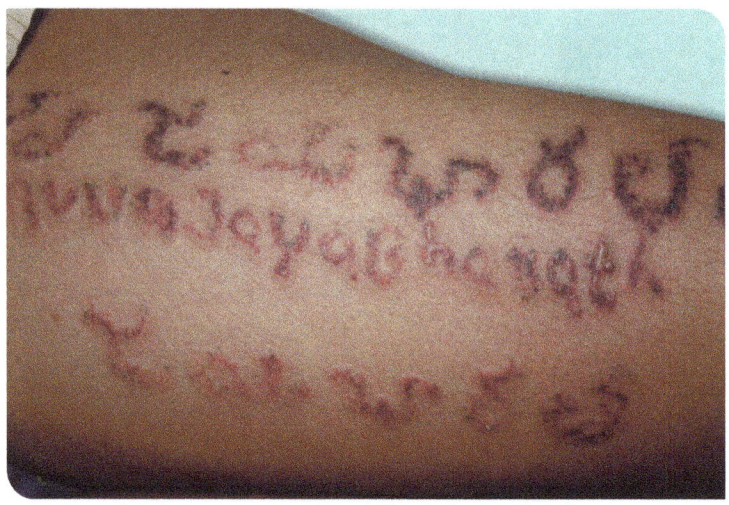

Fig. 7.34: Purpura and petechiae after QS Nd:YAG laser treatment.

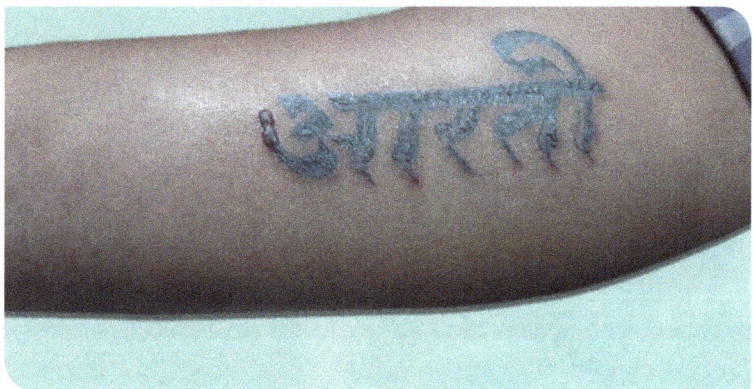

Fig. 7.35: Blistering following QS Nd:YAG laser.

- As already discussed, localized allergic reactions can occur in tattoos, with almost any color ink and can result in urticaria and granulomatous reactions. Mercury-containing red ink is the most common cause for allergic tattoo reactions (Fig. 7.39). Other reactions reported include lichenoid and photoallergic reactions. Cadmium in the yellow ink is known to cause photoallergic reactions. After QS laser treatment, the ink particles may get further mobilized, and trigger a severe allergic response. Systemic allergic reactions may also occur in such patients (Fig. 7.40). Hence, if a patient exhibits a cutaneous reaction within a tattoo, the reaction should be treated with steroid creams and only then should one attempt QS laser treatment with caution. A test patch is always recommended. Patients with persistent allergic reactions in tattoos may be

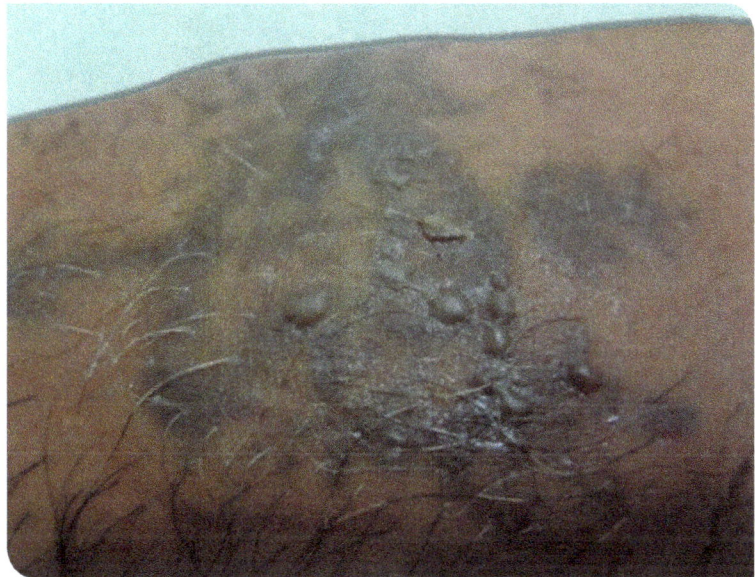

Fig. 7.36: Blistering following QS Nd:YAG laser.
Source: Dr Shashikumar BM.

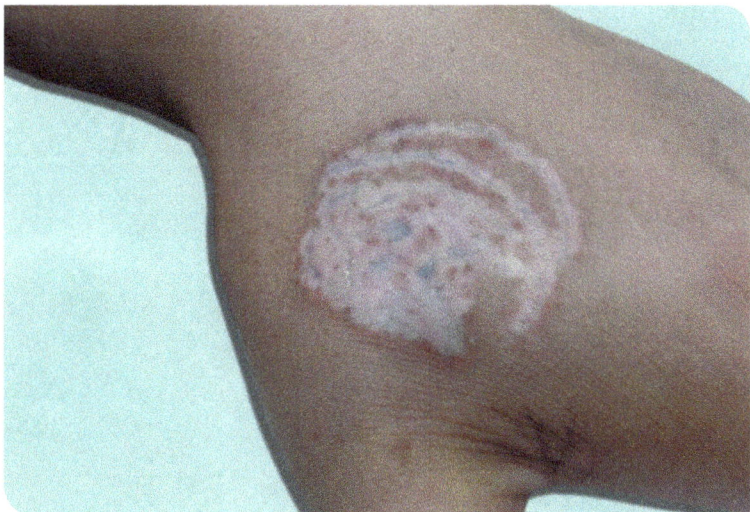

Fig. 7.37: Hypopigmentation following QS Nd:YAG laser.

treated with CO_2 or Er:YAG laser ablation. Anaphylactic reactions are extremely rare but should be kept in mind.

- Scarring may occur if very high fluence is used. A high fluence may result in burns which, if secondarily infected, may lead to scar formation.
- Keloid and hypertrophic scar (Fig. 7.41)

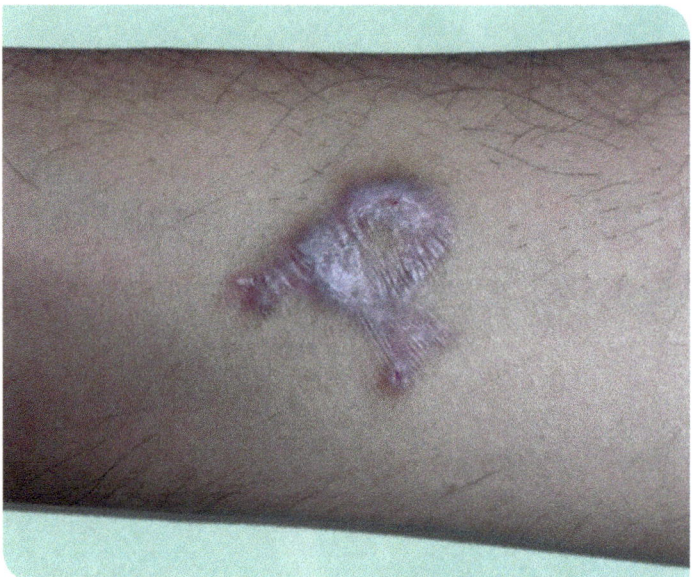

Fig. 7.38: Textural changes.
Source: Dr Shashikumar BM.

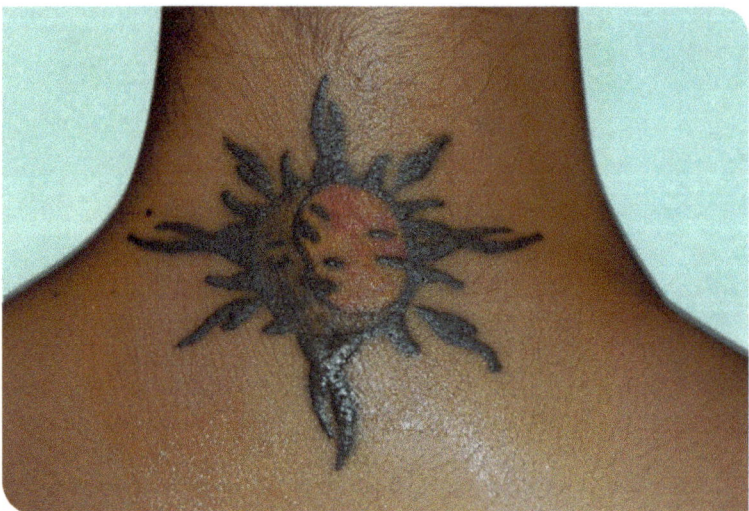

Fig. 7.39: Allergic reaction to tattoo ink.

- Acute compartment syndrome of the upper extremity has been reported following QS 1,064 nm Nd:YAG laser treatment of a decorative tattoo.
- Infection, though uncommon, may occur. An antibiotic ointment and a nonadherent dressing should be applied upon completion of treatment. Patients should be instructed regarding the proper local wound care.

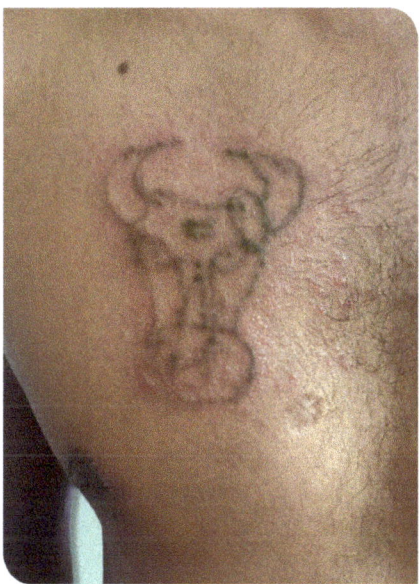

Fig. 7.40: Systemic allergic reaction following Q-switched Nd:YAG laser.
Source: Dr Shashikumar BM.

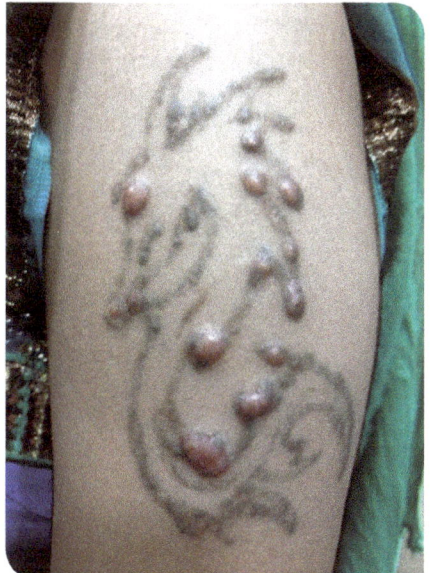

Fig. 7.41: Keloidal scar after third session of laser for tattoo removal.
Source: Dr Savitha AS.

Table 7.2 shows some currently available Q-switched and picosecond lasers.

Table 7.2: Some available Q-switched lasers and picosecond lasers and their specifications.

Laser	Manufacturer	Spot size	Fluence	Repetition rate	Additional features
Spectra XT Q-switched Nd:YAG laser	Lutronic	Up to 10 mm Variable	2J @ 1,064 nm	Up to 10 Hz	Extended platform with 4 wavelengths 1,064 nm, 532 nm, 660 nm, 585 nm
Tri Beam	Jeisys	2–10 mm	1.6J @ 1,064	Up to 20 Hz	5–10 ns pulse duration Dye HP Zoom HP Collimated HP Fractional HP
Helios	Laseroptek	1–7 mm Zoom, 8 mm collimated, 4 x 4 and 5 x 5 fractional	1.3J @ 1,064 nm 0.5J @ 532 nm	Up to 10 Hz	10 ns Pulse duration
Alma-Q	Alma	1–8 mm	1,064–1,200 mj 532–450 mj	10 Hz	Triple mode Q-switched, quasi long pulse and long pulse mode Nd:YAG laser
RevLite and MedLite	Hoya CONBIO-Cynosure	1.2–8.5	Up to 12 J/cm²	10 Hz	Pulse duration 5–20 ns 1,064, 532, 585, 650 nm wavelengths
Discovery Pico	Quanta	2 x 2; 3 x 3; 4 x 4; 5 x 5; 9 x 9 mm², ø 3; 4.5; 6; 7.5; 9; 10.5 mm round; 8 mm fractional round	Pico 800 mj @ 1064 nm Pico 300 mj @ 532 nm	Up to 10 Hz	Q-switched mode pulse duration 6 ns Photothermal mode 300 microsecond 2J
PICOPLUS	Lutronic	1–10 mm, Focused Dots hand piece	Up to 2 J	Up to 10 Hz	Pico- and Nanosecond range Pico Toning 4 wavelengths 532, 1,064, 660, 585 nm
PicoSure	Cynosure	2–6 mm Zoom HP, Fixed HP 6, 8 and 10 mm	Up to 200 mj	10 Hz	755 nm Alex Pico 750 PS Pulse duration
PicoWay	Syneron-Candela	2–10 mm	400 mj @ 1,064 nm 200 mj @ 532 nm	Up to 10 Hz	375–450 PS Pulse duration

CONCLUSION

Tattoo removal with lasers has witnessed a paradigm shift of late. Conventional individual laser sessions are being replaced by multi-pass techniques delivering the equivalent of 2–3 laser sessions that were spaced over weeks and months. Techniques such as R20 and R0 have proved to be effective yet safe even in darker skin types. Combination protocols such as fractional lasers with Q-switched Nd:YAG lasers and picosecond lasers have shown promise aiding faster clearing and improving the safety profile for patients. The availability of laser responsive inks and picosecond lasers has opened new directions wherein someday laser tattoo removal could be possible in a single session!

REFERENCES

1. Buckland AW. "On Tattooing", in Journal of the Royal Anthropological Institute of Great Britain and Ireland. 1887;12:318-28.
2. Aurangabadkar SJ. Shifting paradigm in laser tattoo removal. J Cutan Aesthet Surg. 2015;8:3-4.
3. Goldberg DJ. Pigmented lesions, tattoos, and disorders of hypopigmentation. In: Goldberg DJ (Ed). Laser Dermatology Pearls and Problems, 1st edition. Massachusetts: Blackwell publishing; 2008. pp. 71-114.
4. Shah SD, Aurangabadkar SJ. Newer trends in laser tattoo removal. J Cutan Aesthet Surg. 2015;8:25-9.
5. McClung FJ, Hellwarth RW. Giant optical pulsations from ruby. J Appl Phys. 1962;33:828.
6. Anderson RR, Parrish JA. Selective photothermolysis: precise microsurgery by selective absorption of pulsed radiation. Science. 1983;220:524-7.
7. Polla LL, Margolis RJ, Dover JS, et al. Melanosomes are a primary target of Q-switches ruby laser irradiation in guinea pig skin. J Invest Dermatol. 1987;89:281-6.
8. Ho DD, London R, Zimmerman GB, et al. Laser-tattoo removal—a study of the mechanism and the optimal treatment strategy via computer simulations. Lasers Surg Med. 2002;30:389-97.
9. Kuperman-Beade M, Levine VJ, Ashinoff R. Laser removal of tattoos. Am J Clin Dermatol. 2001;2:21-5.
10. Kilmer SL. Laser eradication of pigmented lesions and tattoos. Dermatol Clin. 2002;20:37-53.
11. Kilmer SL, Garden JM. Laser treatment of pigmented lesions and tattoos. Semin Cutan Med Surg. 2000;19:232-44.
12. Schmults CD, Wheeland RG. Pigmented lesions and tattoos. In: Goldberg DJ, Dover JS, Alam M (Eds). Procedures in Cosmetic Dermatology: Laser and Lights, 1st edition. Philadelphia: Elsevier; 2005. pp. 41-66.
13. Kilmer SL. Laser treatment of tattoos. Dermatol Clin. 1997;15:409-17.
14. Grevelink JM, Duke D, van Leeuwen RL, et al. Laser treatment of tattoos in darkly pigmented patients: efficacy and side effects. J Am Acad Dermatol. 1996;34:653-6.

15. Adrian RM, Griffin L. Laser tattoo removal. Clin Plast Surg. 2000;27:181-92.
16. Barlow RJ, Hruza GJ. Lasers and light tissue interactions. In: Goldberg DJ, Dover JS, Alam M (Eds). Procedures in Cosmetic Dermatology: Laser and Lights, 1st edition. Philadelphia: Elsevier; 2005;1-11.
17. Koay J, Orengo I. Application of local anesthetics in dermatologic surgery. Dermatol Surg. 2002;28:143-8.
18. Drake LA, Dinehart SM, Goltz RW. Guidelines of care for local and regional anesthesia in cutaneous surgery. Guidelines/Outcomes Committee: American Academy of Dermatology. J Am Acad Dermatol. 1995;33(3):504-9.
19. Kilmer SL, Lee MS, Grevelink JM, et al. The Q-switched Nd:YAG laser (1064 nm) effectively treats tattoos. A controlled, dose-response study. Arch Dermatol. 1993;129:971-8.
20. Aurangabadkar S, Mysore V. Standard guidelines of care: lasers for tattoos and pigmented lesions. Indian J Dermatol Venereol Leprol. 2009;75:111-26.
21. Grevelink JM, Duke D, van Leeuwen RL, et al. Laser treatment of tattoos in darkly pigmented patients: efficacy and side effects. J Am Acad Dermatol. 1996;34:653-6.
22. Kilmer SL, Anderson RR. Clinical use of Q-switched ruby and Q-switched Nd:YAG (1064 nm and 532 nm) lasers for treatment of tattoos. J Dermatol Surg Oncol. 1993;19:330-8.
23. Levine VJ, Geronemus RG. Tattoo removal with the Q-switched ruby laser and the Q-switched Nd:YAG laser: a comparative study. Cutis. 1995;55:291-6.
24. Leuenberger ML, Mulas MW, Hata TR, et al. Comparison of the Q-switched alexandrite, Nd:YAG, and ruby lasers in treating blue-black tattoos. Dermatol Surg. 1999;25:10-4.
25. Kilmer SL, Lee MS, Anderson RR. Treatment of multicoloured tattoos with the Q-switched Nd:YAG laser (532 nm): a dose response study with comparison to the Q-switched ruby laser. Lasers Surg Med Suppl. 1993;5:54.
26. Haedersdal M, Bech-Thomsen N, Wulf HC. Skin reflectance-guided laser selections for treatment of decorative tattoos. Arch Dermatol. 1996;132:403-7.
27. Alster TS. Q-switched alexandrite laser treatment (755 nm) of professional and amateur tattoos. J Am Acad Dermatol. 1995;33:69-73.
28. Moreno-Arias GA, Casals-Andreu M, Camps-Fresneda A. Use of Q-switched alexandrite laser (755 nm, 100 ns) for removal of traumatic tattoo of different origins. Laser Surg Med. 1999;25:445-50.
29. Ashinoff R, Geronemus RG. Rapid response of traumatic and medical tattoos to treatment with the QS Ruby laser. Plast Reconstr Surg. 1993;91:841-5.
30. Anderson RR, Geronemus R, Kilmer SL, et al. Cosmetic tattoo ink darkening. A complication of Q-switched and pulsed-laser treatment. Arch Dermatol. 1993;129:1010-4.
31. Ross EV, Yashar S, Michaud N, et al. Tattoo darkening and nonresponse after laser treatment: a possible role for titanium dioxide. Arch Dermatol. 2001;137:33-7.
32. Fusade T, Toubel G, Grognard C, et al. Treatment of gunpowder traumatic tattoo by Q-switched Nd:YAG laser: an unusual adverse effect. Dermatol Surg. 2000;26:1057-9.
33. Taylor CR. Laser ignition of traumatically embedded firework debris. Lasers Surg Med. 1998;22:157-8.
34. Kirby W, Desai A, Desai T, et al. The Kirby-Desai scale: A proposed scale to assess tattoo-removal treatments. J Clin Aesthet Dermatol. 2009;2:32-7.

35. Kossida T, Rigopoulos D, Katsambas A, et al. Optimal tattoo removal in a single laser session based on the method of repeated exposures. J Am Acad Dermatol. 2012;66:271-7.
36. Bunert N, Homey B, Gerber PA. Successful treatment of a professional tattoo with the R20 method. Hautarzt. 2014;65:853-5.
37. Reddy KK, Brauer JA, Anolik R, et al. Topical perfluorodecalin resolves immediate whitening reactions and allows rapid effective multiple pass treatment of tattoos. Lasers Surg Med. 2013;45:76-80.
38. Weiss ET, Geronemus RG. Combining fractional resurfacing with Q-S ruby laser for tattoos. Dermatol Surg. 2010;36:1-3.
39. Marini L, Kozarev J, Grad L, et al. Fractional Er:YAG skin conditioning for enhanced efficacy for Nd:YAG Q switched laser tattoo removal. J Laser Health Acad. 2012;1:35-40.
40. Bencini PL, Cazzaniga S, Tourlaki A, et al. Removal of tattoos by q-switched laser: variables influencing outcome and sequelae in a large cohort of treated patients. Arch Dermatol. 2012;148(12):1364-9.
41. Ross V, Naseef G, Lin G, et al. Comparison of responses of tattoos to picosecond and nanosecond Q-switched neodymium: YAG lasers. Arch Dermatol. 1998;134(2):167-71.
42. Au S, Liolios AM, Goldman MP. Analysis of incidence of bulla formation after tattoo treatment using the combination of the picosecond Alexandrite laser and fractionated CO2 ablation. Dermatol Surg. 2015;41(2):242-5.
43. Brauer JA, Reddy KK, Anolik R, et al. Successful and rapid treatment of blue and green tattoo pigment with a novel picosecond laser. Arch Dermatol. 2012;148(7):820-3.
44. Saedi N, Metelitsa A, Petrell K, et al. Treatment of tattoos with a picosecond alexandrite laser: A prospective trial. Arch Dermatol. 2012;148:1360-3.
45. Elsaie ML, Nouri K, Vejjabhinanta V, et al. Topical imiquimod in conjunction with Nd:YAG laser for tattoo removal. Lasers Med Sci. 2009;24:871-5.
46. Ricotti CA, Colaco SM, Shamma HN, et al. Laser-assisted tattoo removal with topical 5% imiquimod cream. Dermatol Surg. 2007;33:1082-91.
47. Murphy MJ. A novel, simple and efficacious technique for tattoo removal resulting in less pain using the Q-switched Nd:YAG laser. Lasers Med Sci. 2014;29:1445-7.
48. Fox MA, Diven DG, Sra K, et al. Dermal scatter reduction in human skin: A method using controlled application of glycerol. Lasers Surg Med. 2009;41:251-5.
49. Luebberding S, Alexiades-Armenakas M. New tattoo approaches in dermatology. Dermatol Clin. 2014;32:91-6.

Chapter 8

Other Methods of Tattoo Removal

R Raghunatha Reddy, Shilpa K

INTRODUCTION

Tattooing is an invasive procedure in which coloring pigments are introduced into the skin permanently by multiple punctures. Tattoos can be decorative, accidental or sometimes therapeutic. Tattooing has been practiced since ages in different countries and cultures for various reasons. In recent times the number of people seeking tattoos has raised rapidly. A study in United States has shown that 25% of the population aged between 18 years and 50 years have a tattoo.[1,2] Another study has shown these decorative markings are sometimes obtained impulsively, before the age of 18 years or while under the influence of alcohol or recreational drugs,[3] and many eventually regret their decision. With increase in number of patients seeking tattoos, there is also increasing in number of people opting for tattoo removal.

REASON FOR TATTOO REMOVAL

Patients seek tattoo removal for varied reasons:
- Complications arising out of tattoo procedures (Box 8.1), the prevalence of which is approximately 2% to 3%[4]
- Some patients may report feelings of embarrassment, low self-esteem, and stigmatization associated with their tattoos, and may seek removal
- When done under the influence of alcohol or substance abuse, may regret later and seek removal
- In some professions and organizations, like in defense, tattoos are not acceptable.
- Tattoos are forbidden in certain religions
- Due to social beliefs and customs.

Box 8.1: Complications in tattoo procedures.

Infections
- Bacterial:
    - Tetanus, impetigo
    - Skin infection (Methicillin-resistant *Staphylococcus aureus*)
    - Endocarditis
    - Tuberculosis cutis
    - Syphilis
    - Chancroid
    - Sepsis
- Viral:
    - Verruca vulgaris
    - Molluscum contagiosum
    - Human immunodeficiency virus
    - Hepatitis B and C
- Fungal:
    - Superficial and deep fungal infections

Koebnerization
- Psoriasis
- Lichen planus
- Sarcoidosis pyoderma gangrenosum
- Chronic lupus erythematosus
- Vitiligo

Reactions to pigment particles
- Lichenoid reactions
- Granulomatous reactions
- Pseudolymphomatous reaction
- Pseudoepitheliomatous hyperplasia

MILESTONES IN THE HISTORY OF TATTOO REMOVAL TECHNIQUES[5]

Tattoo removal techniques are in practice from pre-historic era. Until 50 years ago, chemical and mechanical methods remained the mainstay of tattoo removal.

In 543 AD, Greek physician Aetius first described the process called "salabrasion", which involves abrading the skin followed by application of salts or other chemicals.[6]

Dermabrasion, in which a wire brush or diamond fraise was used to abrade the skin to remove tattoo pigment within and tattoo itself.

Various other products like trichloroacetic acid and abrasive devices were in use, although their effectiveness and safety were questionable. Use of such non-selective destructive modalities resulted in partial or complete tattoo removal along with risk of scarring and depigmentation.[7]

Simple surgical excision of the skin containing the tattoo has also been an option for a long time. Though it removed the tattoo, it always left a linear scar. Surgical excision followed by skin grafting was another such technique.

In 1960, Maiman created the first laser using a synthetic ruby crystal.[8] Within 3 years, Goldman demonstrated the ability of laser light to selectively destroy chromophore targets in the skin.[9]

In 1967, Goldman and others described successful tattoo removal by both the Q-switched (QS) ruby laser and the QS Nd:YAG (neodymium-doped yttrium aluminum garnet).[10,11] However, the lack of a thorough understanding of the physics at work combined with unpredictable clinical outcomes caused QS lasers to fall out of favor.[12] In the late 1960s and 1970s, continuous lasers such as the carbon dioxide and argon-ion lasers became the treatment of choice for tattoo removal.[13,14]

Then, in the early 1980s, Anderson and Parrish described their groundbreaking theory of selective photothermolysis, in which QS lasers could be used to destroy pigment targets in the skin selectively.[15,16]

LIMITATIONS OF LASER TATTOO REMOVAL

Though the use of lasers is the most popular therapeutic modality with the best aesthetic results, it has certain limitations which include:
- There may be lack of availability and access to LASER
- Requires multiple sittings and removal may take months
- Certain colors like red and yellow are resistant
- Removal may be incomplete and may leave a ghost images
- Over all treatment is expensive
- In special circumstances, like the name tattoos which needs to be removed completely for various reasons. LASERS may not be able to do that and hence the need for complete removal by surgical methods despite the fact that they produce scar.

SURGICAL TECHNIQUES FOR TATTOO REMOVAL

These techniques are "mechanical" which include salabrasion, dermabrasion, and surgical excision with primary closure or followed by grafting. Though the first method is currently abandoned, dermabrasion in combination with other technique is done less frequently.

Excision

Punch Excision

Small circular tattoos commonly found on forehead, chin, and forearm can be excised using skin biopsy punches.

Procedure: After preparing the parts, the skin is stretched perpendicular to the direction of relaxed skin tension line (RSTL), an appropriate sized punch which can completely remove the tattoo is kept perpendicular to skin, and with slow twisting back and forth movements it is advanced till the subcutis (where we get a giveaway feel). The tissue is then held with forceps and cut at the base. This technique often allows the wound to rest along RSTL and wound closed with appropriate suture material of the size 5-0 or 6-0 depending on the size (Figs. 8.1A and B). Wound dressed followed by suture removal on 5th to 7th day depending on the site.

Precautions: Tattoos of up to 4 mm size can be removed with punch excision. Closure of punch excision above 4 mm in size often cause dog ear, thus causing less than optimal cosmesis compared to small ellipse.[17] Using larger punches (>6 mm) can result in dog ear formation which require further correction resulting in lengthier scar. In such circumstances, elliptical excision will be a better option in such condition or alternately the defect may be closed with full-thickness skin grafting of 1 mm larger size donor skin harvested from postauricular area.

Elliptical Excision

The elliptical (fusiform) excision is a basic tool of cutaneous surgery due to ease of construction in the ensuing suture line along the RSTLs with good aesthetic outcomes. Elliptical variations are easily designed and can be adapted to many situations.[18] Linear tattoos along RSTL commonly found on forearm and neck can be excised with simple elliptical excision and closure.

Planning and procedure: An ideal ellipse is the one in which the length and width ratio is 3:1 and the angle between the two limbs is 30°. However slight modification can be done according to the size and site of tattoos. After drawing an ellipse, incision line is put over the pre-marked lines. Then the tattooed skin is dissected at the level of mid-dermis and excised. After excision proper undermining has to be done on both sides and wound has to be closed in two layers with buried intradermal and percutaneous sutures to reduce tension on suture line. Compression dressing has to be put and patient should be advised to avoid vigorous movements or weight lifting in the operated area. Suture removal done from 7th (face) to 10th day (forearms) depending on the site (Figs. 8.2A to D).

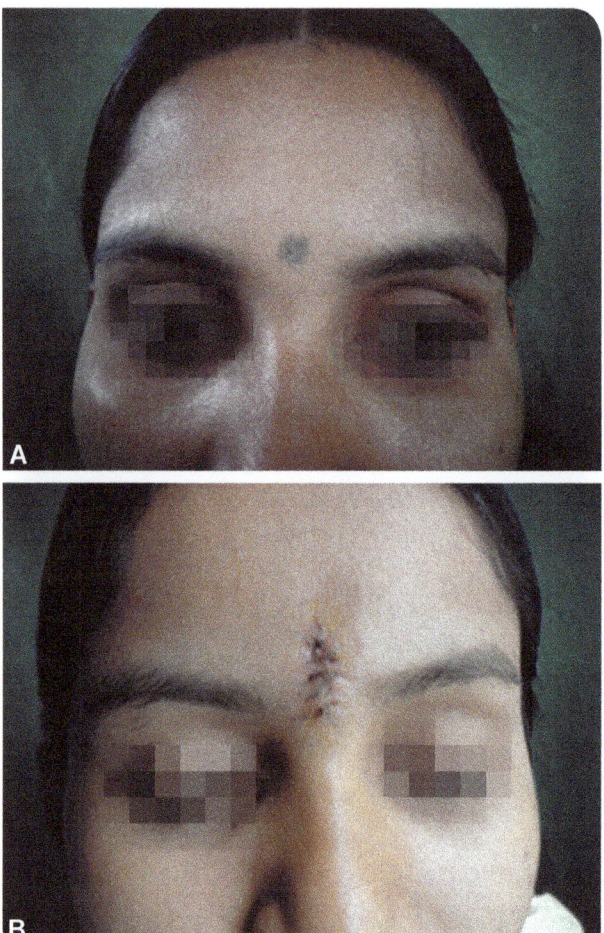

Figs. 8.1A and B: (A) A circular tattoo on forehead; (B) After punch excision and closure.

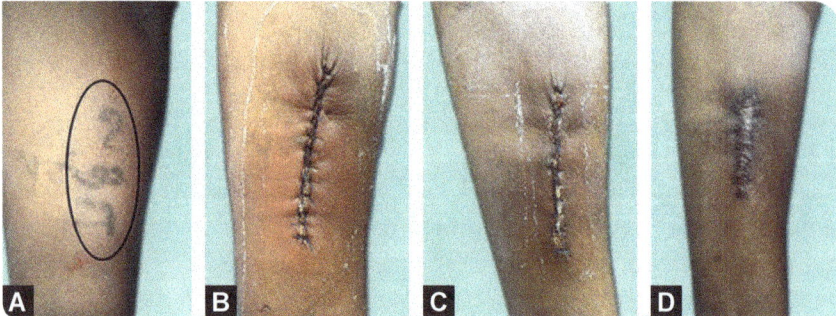

Figs. 8.2A to D: (A) Tattoo on forearm with elliptical excision planned; (B) Immediately after excision and primary closure, note the tension in the wound; (C) On the third day, minimal gaping; (D) A bad linear scar after a month with poor results.

Precautions: A linear tattoo of width up to 2 to 3 cm depending on the laxity of skin can be excised and closed primarily. A wider tattoo may require serial excision in two to three sittings. Primary closure of wider tattoos may result in excess tension on suture line, wound gaping and a bad scar. Proper undermining and wound closure in layers reduces the tension along suture line. The most important point during skin closure is to keep wound sutured edges slightly everted in order to overcome the spreading of scar which is inevitable to occur in due course of time. Wound edge eversion improves with time.

S-plasty

S-plasty is a modification of elliptical excision in which an S-shaped curvilinear incision instead of a straight line incision is made to reduce tension and improve healing in areas where the skin is loose.

Planning and procedure: The planning is similar to elliptical excision; however, the edges of an elliptical excision are modified in the shape of letter "S" which realigns along RSTL of extremities. Further procedure like excision, undermining, and wound closure is similar to elliptical excision and closure. However, line of closure will be S-shaped rather than linear closure of elliptical closure, which may help to break the monotony associated with linear straight line scar (Figs. 8.3A and B).

Advantage: This technique further reduces tension on suture line. It also prevents dog ear formation and thus reduces the length of the scar line.[19] It is suitable for linear tattoos of forearm.

Serial Excision

Serial or staged skin excision is a time-honored technique that was first described by Morestin in 1915 and later, independently, by Sinstrunk in 1926. A wider tattoo which cannot be removed completely with either elliptical or S-plasty can be removed with serial excision.

Principle: The principle relies on the fact that there is "creep" (relaxation) of the tensioned skin over time. This relaxation is initially "mechanical" due to uncoiling of elastin fibers and reorientation of collagen fibers in the direction of the strain, and later is followed by "biological" creep due to remodeling of the skin. This biological creep allows the skin once more to undergo "mechanical" creep.[20]

Planning and procedure: In serial excision technique, a part of tattoo either in the center or edge is removed in the first stage as in elliptical or S-shaped excision technique described above in Figures 8.1A and B. The remaining part of the tattoo will be excised after 6–10 weeks. In this way the entire tattoo can be removed in 2–4 surgical sessions (Figs. 8.4A to F).

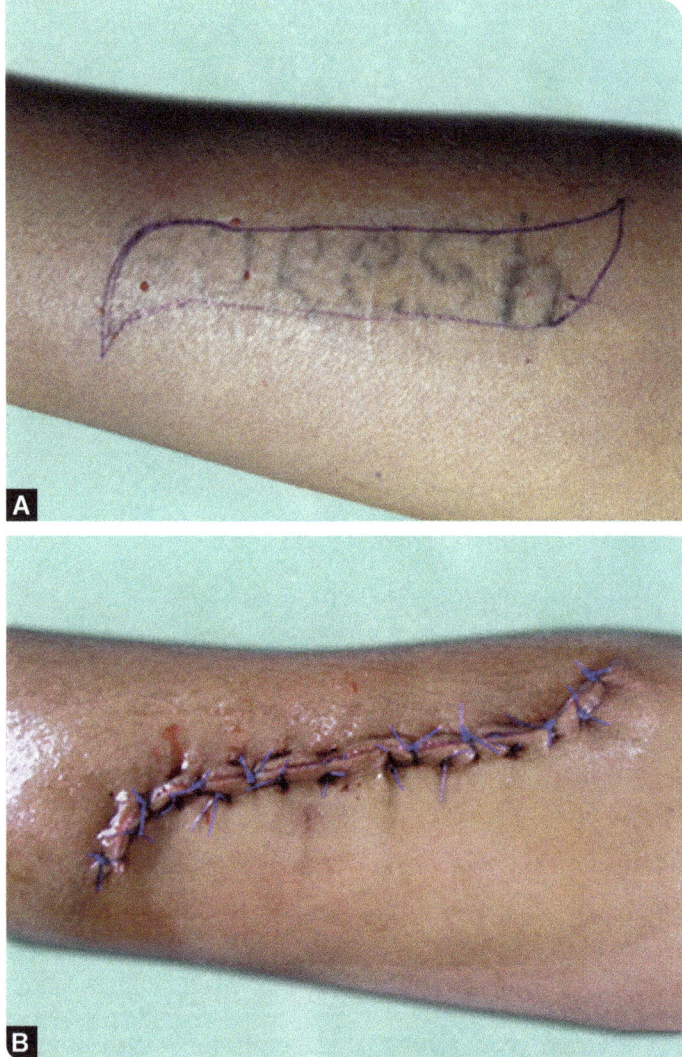

Figs. 8.3A and B: (A) Tattoo on forearm with planned S-shaped excision; (B) Wound closed with S-shaped suture line, immediate postoperative period.

Advantage of serial excision is that the resultant scar can be made to orient along RSTL for a better cosmetic outcome. Tension on the wound edges and thus ensuing bad scar can be avoided. Bigger tattoos may require 2–3 sittings.

Excision followed by Split-thickness Skin Graft

Excision followed by split-thickness skin grafting is a simple means of tattoo removal with very acceptable cosmetic results.

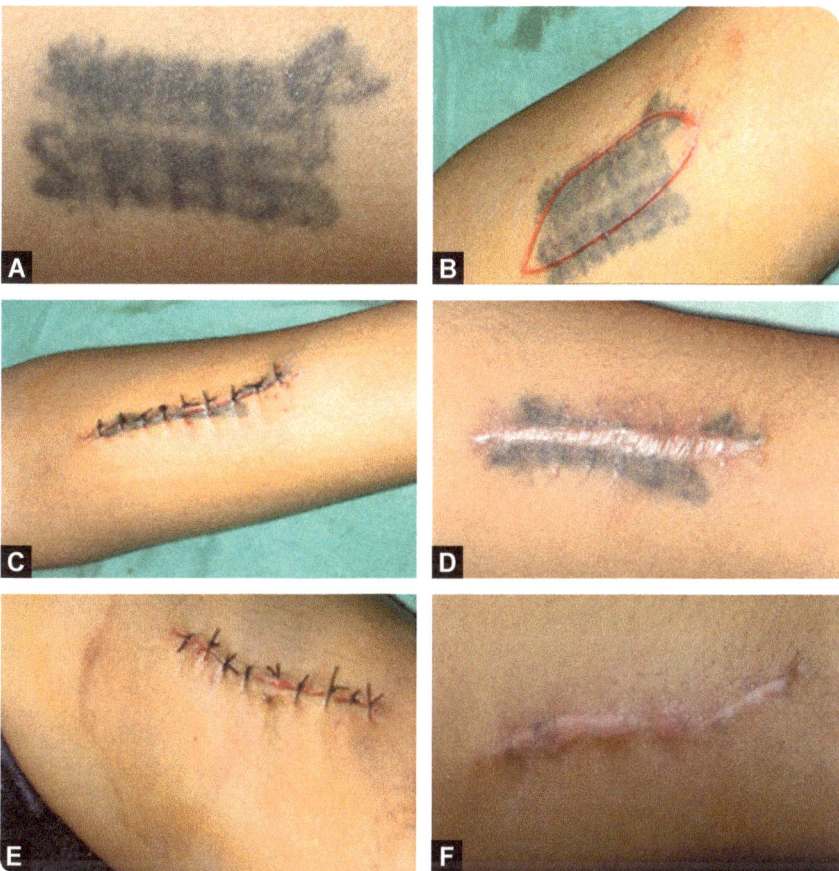

Figs. 8.4A to F: (A) A wide tattoo on forearm; (B) Partial excision in the center; (C) Immediately after first excision; (D) Linear scar along with remnant of tattoo after first stage of excision; (E) Second-stage excision after 12 weeks with complete tattoo removal; and (D) Complete removal with a linear hypertrophic scar.

Procedure and planning: Procedure is done under local anesthesia. Tattooed skin is excised at the level of upper dermis or mid-dermis depending on the level of pigment in the dermis, so that the tattoo pigments are completely removed. Donor area is usually the covered areas like upper thigh or buttocks. After anaesthetizing the part, partial or split-thickness skin graft is harvested using Humby's knife or dermatomes. Skin is stretched by giving traction. Humby's knife is introduced at 45° to skin surface. After reaching the desired depth, Humby's knife is kept parallel to skin and with to and fro movement knife is advanced to get the desired length of the graft. The size of the graft should be kept 10% more than the defect to compensate for the elastic recoil and shrinking of graft. The obtained graft is then placed over the defect. Graft is secured with suture or staples followed by pressure dressing (Figs. 8.5A to F).

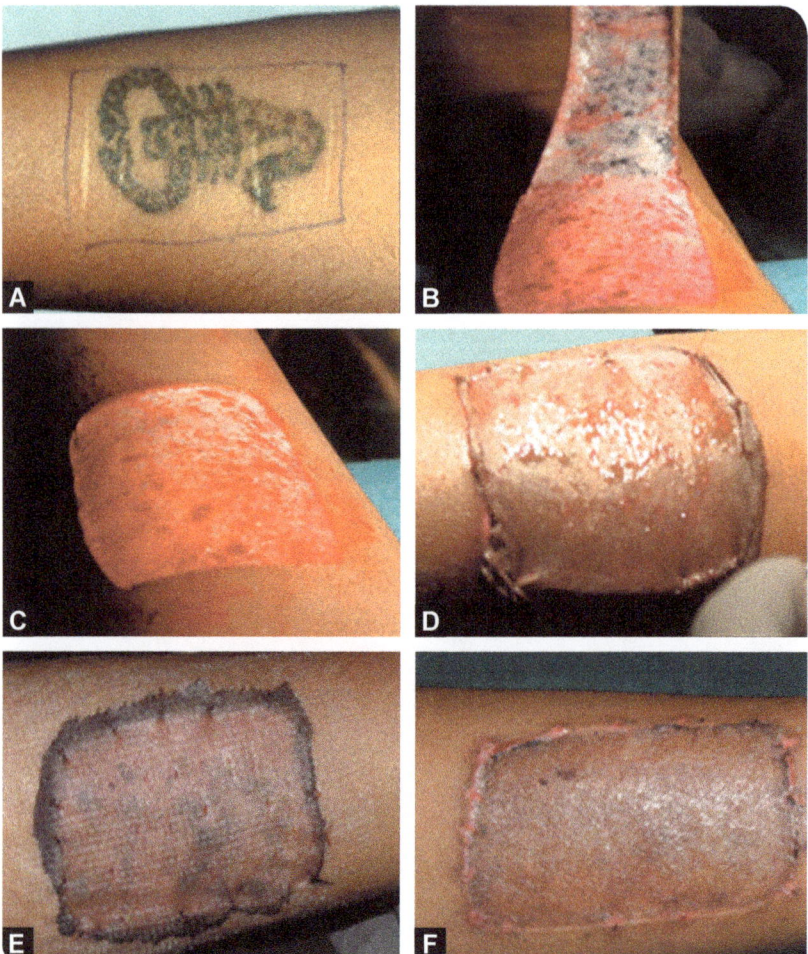

Figs. 8.5A to F: (A) A wide tattoo in forearm; (B) Tattooed area being removed with dissection of skin in the mid-dermis level; (C) Complete removal of tattooed skin; (D) Placing split-thickness graft; (E) Graft secured with suture; and (F) Complete take up of graft with good aesthetic outcome within 6 weeks.

The technique has several advantages: (1) ensures complete removal of tattoo pigments; (2) scar formation is negligible; (3) the procedure may be carried out rapidly, is inexpensive for patients and conserves time for physicians, since it is one-stage procedure compared to serial partial excision.

The disadvantages of this technique include: (1) it gives a stuck on appearance, donor area scarring or depigmentation, and (2) it also requires skill to obtain appropriate grafts.

Modification of the technique is that instead of split skin grafts the defects can also be covered with grafting of autologous and allogenic cultured epithelium after excision of tattoos.[21]

COMPLICATIONS OF SURGICAL EXCISION

Reported complications include difficulties in suturing of the skin, with risk of delayed healing, development of hypertrophic scars, keloids or anatomical distortions resulting in scars less aesthetically acceptable. Permanent scars will result and this should be explained very carefully before treatment. Scars may be red and raised for up to 3 months and then gradually improve over a year to 18 months. In a situation of wide or hypertrophic scar, the scar can be improved with fractional CO_2 laser resurfacing in multiple sittings of 5–6 times 4 weeks apart, which will improve the ensuing scar greatly for better aesthetic results.[22]

Salabrasion

Since ages physicians have tried to remove tattoos without leaving a scar. Aetius (543 AD) was the first to describe the use of salt and chemicals for the purpose.[5,23] Klovekorn (1935) described the abrasion of skin with table salt in order to remove tattoo pigment;[6,24] and Crittenden recently confirmed these results and named the process salabrasion.[25]

Procedure: The tattooed area to be treated is prepared and anesthetized. The patient is then instructed to wrap a moist 4 × 4 gauze sponge impregnated with salt around his index and middle fingers and to begin rubbing the tattoo he wishes to remove. The abrasion continues till the skin becomes "blood" red and appears like good granulation tissue. This usually takes 30–40 minutes. At this point, the treated area is covered with antibiotic ointment and a sterile dressing which is left in place for 3 days. When a dermabrador or tattoo gun is used, the skin is either superficially abraded or punctured in the desired areas and then covered with a layer of table salt. The insult to the dermis must be very superficial. At this point, when the treated area will look raw but not blood red, it is covered with a layer of salt for 4 hours.

Postoperative care: The dressing is then changed and the wound cleaned and redressed with an antibiotic ointment for an additional 3 days. This salted area separates between the 7th and 12th postoperative days. With eschar separation one may see that about half of the ink has been removed. Still more ink leaves the treated area in exudate while the skin is healing. The skin heals quickly and with virtually no scarring. A second treatment can be administered 6–8 weeks after the first. This technique is obsolete now.

Superficial Dermabrasion

Boo-Chai reported that superficial dermabrasion of tattoos creates an inflammatory response and thus promotes the "biologic removal" of pigment through the lymphatics and the sloughing of superficial macrophages.[26] Clabaugh postulated that the pigment-laden phagocytes may become mobile and migrate to the wound surface where they are removed by daily dressing changes.[27] However, the dermabrasion is the prime stimulus for pigment effluvium from the wound; and the postoperative application of gentian violet 2% (Figs. 8.6A to D), triamcinolone acetonide 0.1% lotion, hydrogen peroxide solution 3%, and daily dressing changes in any combination do not significantly increase the amount of pigment removed. Tattoos treated postoperatively without any topical medication responded with pigment loss equal to those treated by any of several other combinations.[28] Trichloroacetic acid is a chemical cauterant that coagulates the proteins of the skin and has been utilized for therapeutic treatment of dermatological conditions.[1] It has also been proposed as a tattoo removal agent.[29,30] However, as the concentration increases, the depth of dermal damage also increases.

CONCLUSION

In LASER era also, surgery still remains as an alternative method of tattoos removal. It remains the first-line choice for small tattoos localized on areas

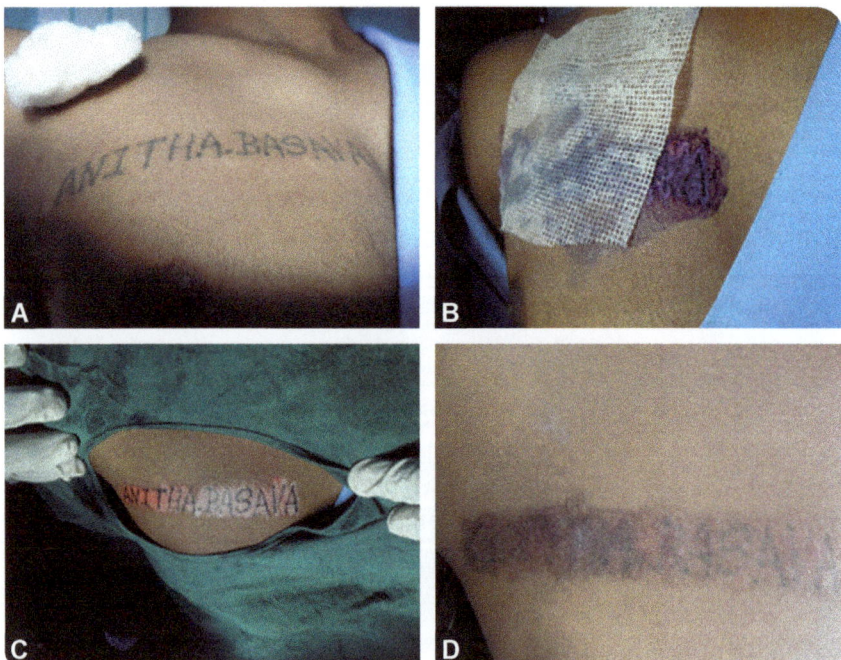

Figs. 8.6A to D: (A) Tattoo on the chest; (B) Immediately after superficial dermabrasion; (C) Everyday dressing with paraffin dressings; (D) After healing with slight hyperpigmentation.

of appropriate laxity. Postoperative scar is all the more discreet and aesthetically pleasing when planned and executed well on an area of significant laxity. Surgery ensures complete excision of the tattoo in one surgical time for smaller tattoos and for wider tattoos a complete excision requires two operative times with a higher risk of vicious scars.

REFERENCES

1. Laumann AE, Derick AJ. Tattoos and body piercings in the United States: a national data set. J Am Acad Dermatol. 2006;55:413-42.
2. Armstrong M, Roberts A, Owen D, et al. Contemporary college students and body piercing. J Adolesc Health. 2004;35(1):58-61.
3. Laumann A, Derick A. Tattoos and body piercings in the United States: a national data set. J Am Acad Dermatol. 2006;55(3):413-21.
4. Michael Urdang, Jennifer T Mallek, William K Mallon, et al. Tattoos and Piercings: A Review for the Emergency Physician. West J Emerg Med. 2011;12(4):393-8.
5. Kathryn M Kent, Emmy M Graber. Laser Tattoo Removal: A Review. Dermatol Surg. 2012;38:1-13.
6. Manchester G. Tattoo removal. A new simple technique. Calif Med. 1973;118(3):10-2.
7. Bernstein E. Laser tattoo removal. Semin Plast Surg. 2007;21(3):175-92.
8. Maiman T. Stimulated optical radiation in ruby. Nature. 1960;187:493-4.
9. Goldman L, Blaney D, Kindel DJ, et al. Effect of the laser beam on the skin. Preliminary report. J Invest Dermatol. 1963;40:121-2.
10. Goldman L, Rockwell R, Meyer R, et al. Laser treatment of tattoos. A preliminary survey of three year's clinical experience. JAMA. 1967;201(11):841-4.
11. Yules R, Laub D, Honey R, et al. The effect of Q-switched ruby laser radiation on dermal tattoo pigment in man. Arch Surg. 1967;95(2):179-80.
12. Glenn Lubeck, Ervin Epstein. Complications of Tattooing. California Medicine. 1952;76(2):83-5.
13. Reid R, Muller S. Tattoo removal by CO laser dermabrasion. Plast Reconstr Surg. 1980;65(6):717-28.
14. Apfelberg D, Maser M, Lash H. Argon laser treatment of decorative tattoos. Br J Plast Surg. 1979;32(2):141-4.
15. Anderson R, Parrish J. Microvasculature can be selectively damaged using dye lasers: a basic theory and experimental evidence in human skin. Lasers Surg Med. 1981;1(3):263-76.
16. Anderson R, Parrish J. Selective photothermolysis: precise microsurgery by selective absorption of pulsed radiation. Science. 1983;220(4596):524-7.
17. Geisse JK. Biopsy techniques for pigmented lesions of skin. Pathology State of Art Reviews. 1994;2(2):181-93. California Society of Pathologists. Philadelphia, Hanley and Belfus inc.
18. Goldberg LH, Murad Alam. Variations and the Eccentric Parallelogram. Elliptical Excisions. Arch Dermatol. 2004;140:176-80.
19. Liu H, Yu N, Shi J, et al. A New Modified S-plasty for Skin Defect Closure. Aesthetic Plast Surg. 2015;39(1):100-5.
20. Paul Roblin. (2016). Optimisation of serial excision. [online] Available from http://docslide.net/documents/optimisation-of-serial-excision.html [Accessed April 2017].

21. Kumagai N. Grafting of autologous and allogenic cultured epithelium after excision of tattoos. Eur J Plast Surg. 1994;17:312.
22. Morgan BD. Aspects of Plastic Surgery. Brit Med J. 1974;6:34-6.
23. Scutt RWB. The chemical removal of tattoos. Br J P Surg. 1972;25:189-94.
24. Kloevekorn GH. Eine einfache methode der entferlung von taetowierungen. Dermatologische Wochenscrhrift. 1935;101:1271.
25. Crittenden FM. Salabrasion-removal of tattoos by superficial abrasion with table salt. Cutis. 1971;7:295-300.
26. Boo-Chai K. The decorataive tattoo—its removal by dermabrasion. Plastic Reconstr Surg. 1963;32:559-63.
27. Clabaugh W. Removal of tattoos by superficial dermabrasion. Arch Dermatol. 1968;98:515-21.
28. Donald Hagerman R, Cranmer LG, Bartok WR, et al. Topical Medications on Dermabraded Tattoos. Arch Dermatol. 1970;102(4):438-9.
29. Hudson D, Lechtape-Gruter R. A simple method of tattoo removal. S Afr Med J. 1990;78(12):748-9.
30. Piggot T, Norris R. The treatment of tattoos with trichloroacetic acid: experience with 670 patients. Br J Plast Surg. 1988;41(2):112-7.

Chapter 9

Tattoo Alternatives

Kavya M

INTRODUCTION

Tattooing for cosmetic purposes has become quite popular in recent times. There are many reasons for which people get tattooed on themselves like for attention seeking purpose or they may be motivated by adventure, artistry or religion. But eventually people want to get rid of tattoos due to various reasons like they want to get rid of ex flame's name/initials or maybe they are not satisfied with the design, etc. They do not realize that removal of tattoo is very tedious and prolonged procedure and is quite expensive than getting a tattoo itself. Also permanent tattoos are prone for adverse effects like allergic reactions to dyes, keloids and risk of infections. Hence as the saying says "Think before you get inked", there is an urgent need for tattoo alternatives. The advantages of temporary tattoos are:

- There is no pain as there is no piercing with needles
- No risk of infection transmission
- Can be removed easily without any traces.

HENNA

Henna, the dried and powdered leaf of *Lawsonia inermis*, is widely used as a dye for the skin, hair, and nails, and as an expression of body art, especially in Islamic and Hindu cultures. As it stains the skin reddish-brown, it is also called "red henna". Many of these cultures believe that henna is good luck and adorn themselves with intricate henna designs in order to denote beauty or joy. Henna tattoos have also become increasingly popular in western countries as the short-term alternative to permanent tattoos. Henna tattoos (Fig. 9.1) are usually harmless but some types of henna can cause powerful allergic reactions.

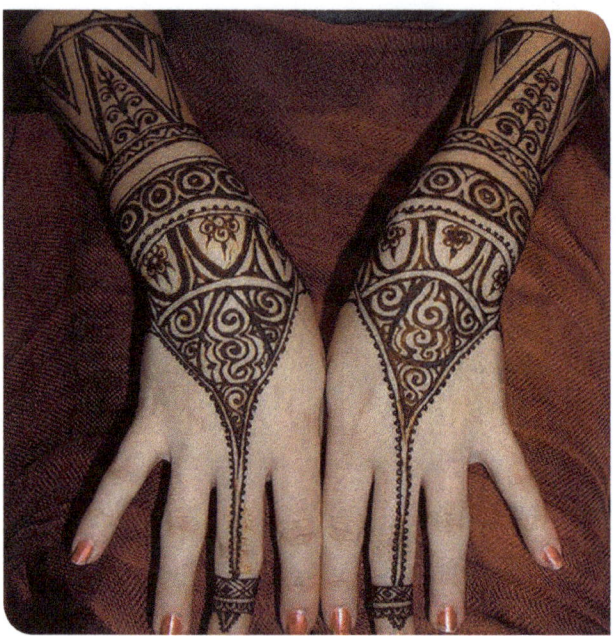

Fig. 9.1: Henna tattoo.

Henna is a vegetable dye that can be brown, red or green. It is actually the dried and powdered leaf of the dwarf evergreen shrub *Lawsonia inermis*. Henna or *Lawsonia inermis* grows throughout Africa, Asia and parts of Australia. Some people refer to it as "Egyptian Privet". Its use dates all the way back to the Bronze Age and ancients celebrated battle victories by adorning themselves and even some of their animals with henna tattoos.

To create the henna tattoo, a paste is made by adding water or oil to henna powder or to ground fresh henna leaves. Essential oils like eucalyptus oil or clove oil, lemon juice, tannin concentrates from brewing tea leaves, coffee powder, sugar, etc. are added to enhance the color. This paste is applied to the skin and allowed to remain there for a minimum of 30 minutes to 2–6 hours as the plant's dye penetrates the skin; the longer the exposure, the darker the color will be. The dried paste is then removed to reveal an orange stain, which will darken over the next 2–4 days. A temporary henna tattoo should last for approximately 2–6 weeks, until the outer layer of the skin exfoliates, depending on skin type, the area of application, sun exposure, and other factors such as bathing and activity level.[1]

When applied to the skin, hair, or nails, the pigment lawsone (2-hydroxy-1,4-naphthoquinone; CI 75480; Natural Orange 6), which is present at a concentration of less than 2% in henna leaves and natural henna preparations, interacts with the keratin therein to give them a reddish-brown (rust-red) color; therefore, a frequently used synonym is "red henna".

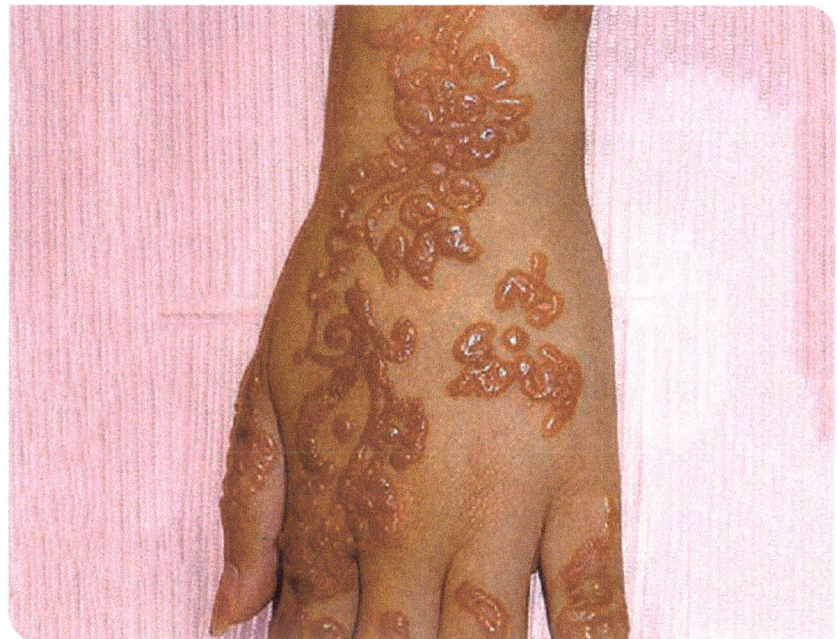

Fig. 9.2: Contact dermatitis to red henna tattoo.

Side Effects of Red Henna

Red henna appears to be generally safe, with only few reports of contact allergy as shown in Figure 9.2 despite its widespread use especially in India. Most of the patients have showed positive patch with henna preparations. The allergen identified in henna is lawsone, but this has been proved only in few studies.[2,3] Thus, the contact allergy may be due to other ingredients of the plant or substances added later, for example, essential oils.[4]

Type I hypersensitivity reactions have been reported in few cases, especially in hair dressers due to inhalation of henna powder as a result of occupational hazard. Type I mediated reactions like sneezing, conjunctivitis, running nose, dry cough, dyspnea, swelling of the face, or generalized urticarial rashes have been reported. The diagnosis is made by prick testing with henna solutions.

Other very rare side effects of henna include problems with peripheral venous cannulation due to heavy floral patterns on both forearms and hands.[5] The structure and redox potential of lawsone (2-hydroxy-1,4-naphthoquinone) are similar to those of 1,4-naphthoquinone, a metabolite of naphthalene and a potent oxidant of glucose-6-phosphate dehydrogenase (G6PD)-deficient cells. Hence, topical application of henna paste may cause life-threatening hemolysis in children with glucose-6-phosphate dehydrogenase deficiency.[6]

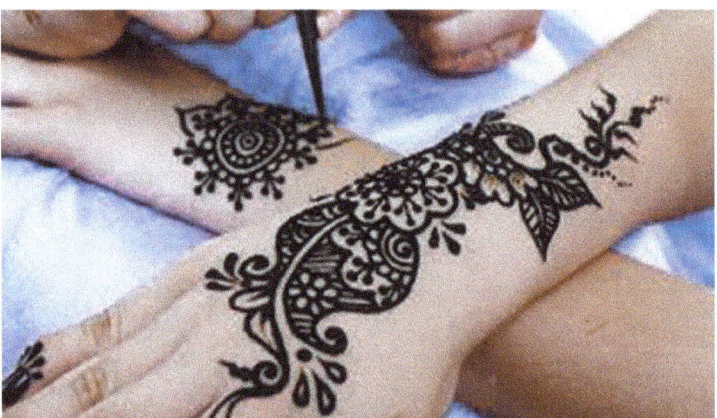

Fig. 9.3: Black henna tattoo.

TEMPORARY BLACK HENNA TATTOO

Black henna is the combination of red henna with p-phenylenediamine (PPD), and is used for temporary "black henna tattoos" (Fig. 9.3). It is also known as skin painting or pseudotattooing.

The term "black henna" is sometimes used to indicate the powder of bush, *Indigofera argentea* (of the Fabaceae family), which is a distinct botanical species.[7] PPD is added to henna to accelerate the dyeing and drying process (to only 30 minutes), to strengthen and darken the color, to enhance the design pattern of the tattoo, and to make the tattoo last longer. These tattoos stain the skin black, and have the appearance of a real tattoo. Black henna can be distinguished from red henna in that it is dark brown or black, does not change color when moistened, and is fixed on the skin in less than 1 hour. In contrast, pure red henna is green–gray in color, tends to turn orange when moistened, and needs between 2 hours and 12 hours to be fixed on the skin.

Paraphenylenediamine is a powerful allergen and is responsible for most of the complications reported after henna tattoos: localized or generalized contact dermatitis, hypertrophic or keloid scars, and temporary or permanent hyper- or hypopigmentation. More rarely, type I hypersensitivity reactions (urticaria, angioedema, or anaphylaxis) with potentially lethal outcomes have been reported. PPD allergy can induce cross-reactivity with other substances, such as hair dyes and textile azo dyes.[8]

ACRYLIC PAINT/SPRAY

Acrylic paint can be used as a temporary tattoo which can be applied with brush with a little bit of water. It dries in minutes and lasts for 4–5 hours.

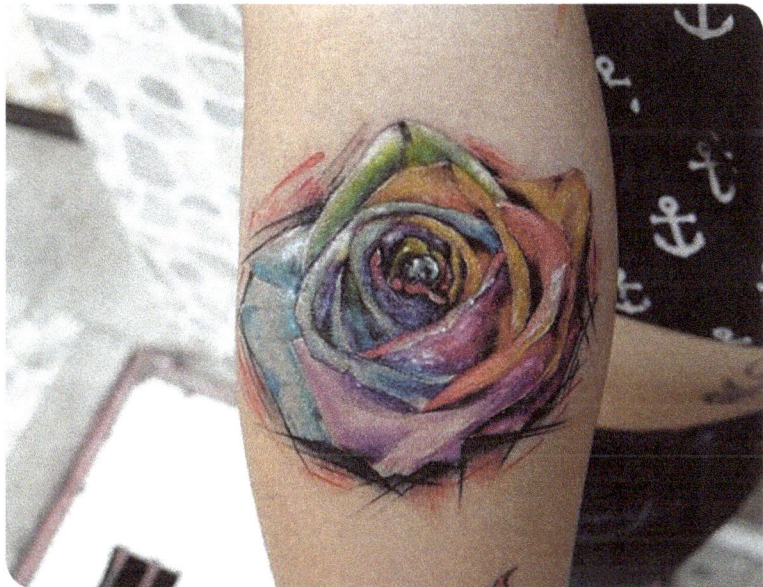

Fig. 9.4: Acrylic paint tattoo.

The main limitation is cracking and the paint is not waterproof. Figure 9.4 depicts acrylic paint tattoo.

LIQUID EYELINER/PENCILS

Waterproof liquid eyeliner is one of the best options for temporary tattoo, as the ink will last longer and is less prone to smudging during sweating or when it gets wet. Alternatively, eyeliner pencils can also be used. With pencils we can vary the pressure to create shading effect on our skin. With the eyeliners, precise and bold strokes can be done as shown in Figure 9.5. It can be easily removed with oil-based make up removers without leaving any traces.

SKIN SAFE INKS

India ink is a nontoxic simple black or colored ink used in art world for drawing and outlining especially in comics and calligraphy. It is mainly used for homemade tattoos since it is easily available and inexpensive. Basic India ink is made up of fine soot, known as lampblack which is combined in water to form a liquid. The carbon molecules are in colloidal suspension and form a waterproof layer after drying. Binding agents such as gelatin or shellac is added to make the ink more durable once dried. The tattoo lasts for 4–5 hours.

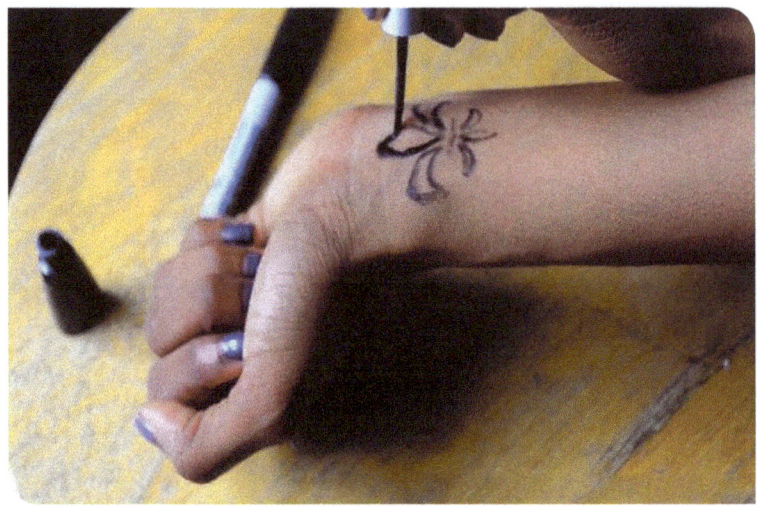

Fig. 9.5: Temporary tattoo with liquid eyeliner.

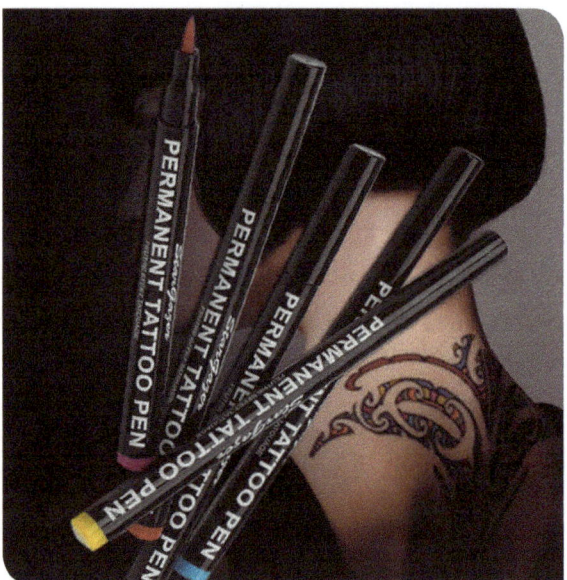

Fig. 9.6: Tattoo pen/markers.

TATTOO PEN/MARKERS

The Tattoo pen was first developed by Tim Hendricks in the United States of America. It was the only pen which was meant for drawing directly onto the skin for pre-tattoo purposes. But nowadays many markers are available in the market (Fig. 9.6 shows one of the markers and tattoo done with the

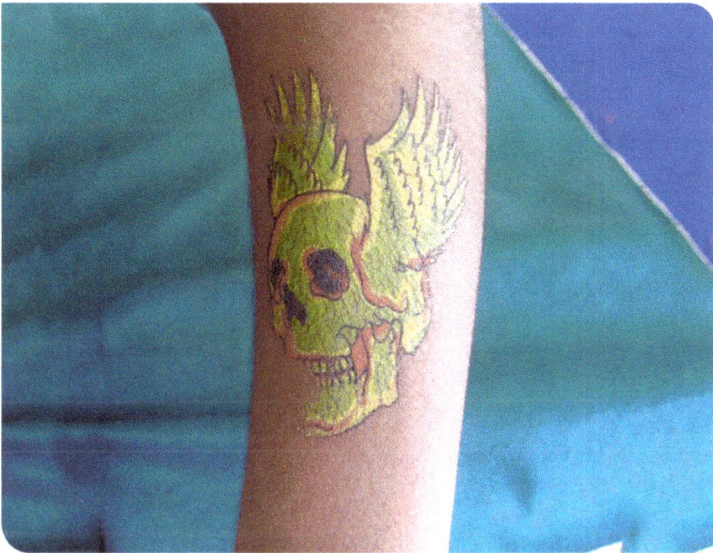

Fig. 9.7: Decal tattoos.

pen). They are available in different colors. The thin tip of the marker pens allows for perfect drawings of thin and thick lines. The color lasts for 24 hours' duration and it does not smudge. It can be removed with corrector or make up remover.

DECAL TEMPORARY TATTOOS

The most popular temporary tattoos especially among children are these press-on decal or water transfer tattoos. The tattoo is printed on a water permeable paper. The tattoo should be placed on the body with the ink-side down and water is applied on the paper. The image transfers to the body surface on contact with the water as shown in Figure 9.7. Only pigments used in cosmetics that are approved by Food and Drug Administration (FDA) are used in these tattoos, so they are nontoxic and nonallergenic. But in recent days the tattoos manufactured in China and Taiwan include nonapproved pigments that can cause allergic reaction. The tattoo usually lasts for a day or up to a week. They can be easily removed with rubbing alcohol or baby oil.

FOIL/FLASH METALLIC TEMPORARY TATTOOS

These are variation of decal-style temporary tattoos. These tattoos have metallic shine of gold/silver in them (Fig. 9.8). Hence, they are popular in wedding parties. They look similar to permanent tattoos but with more flexibility.

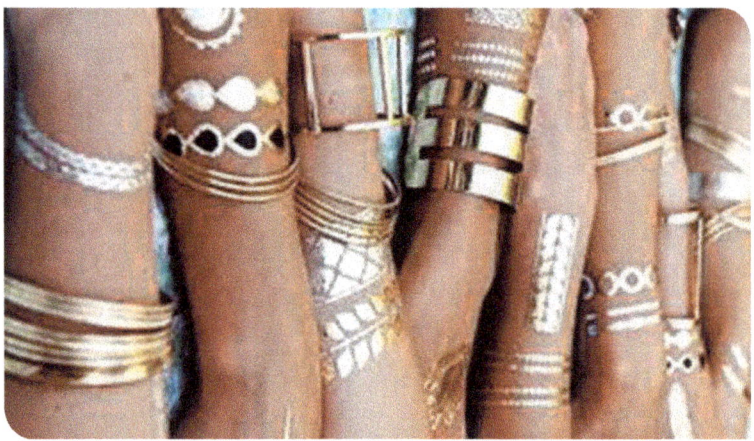

Fig. 9.8: Foil/Flash tattoos with metallic shine.

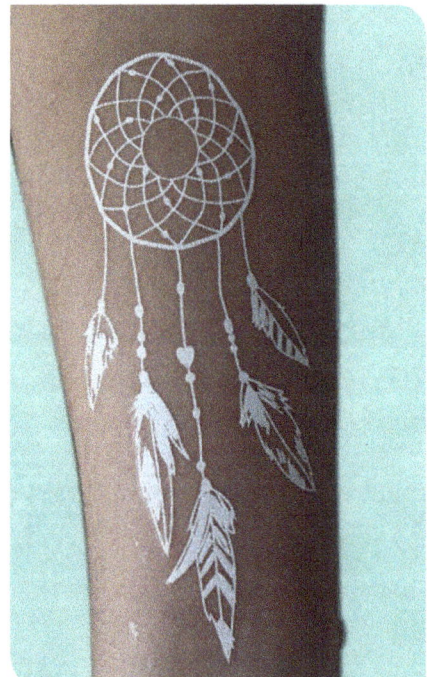

Fig. 9.9: White lace tattoos.

WHITE LACE TATTOOS

These are decal tattoos available in sheets. Also known as "white henna tattoos" (Fig. 9.9). They are in trend especially during summers. Lasts for a week and can be removed easily.

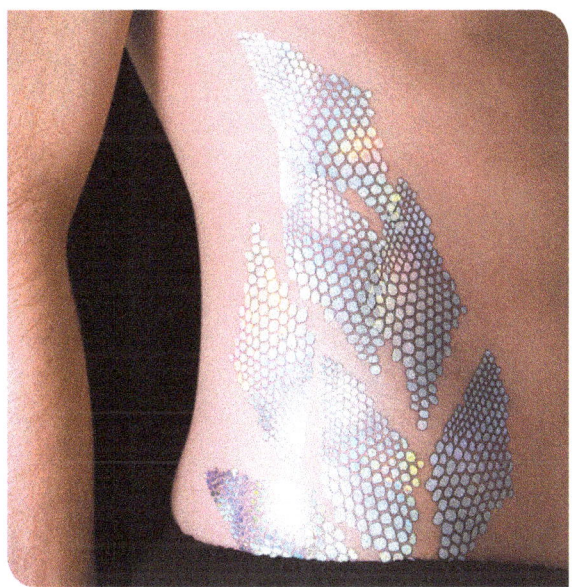

Fig. 9.10: Fish scale holographic tattoo.

HOLOGRAPHIC TEMPORARY TATTOOS

These are temporary tattoos which are rainbow-colored and have iridescent effect. They change color depending on the sunlight and even glow in the dark shown in Figure 9.10 is fish scale tattoo. This property makes them different from regular foil tattoos. They are popular in younger generations and are fun to wear in parties. They usually stay for 5–7 days.

UV TATTOOS/BLACK-LIGHT TATTOOS

They are popularly known as glow in the dark tattoos. But there is difference in both of these tattoos. The glow in the dark tattoos (Fig. 9.11) is made of phosphorous, which is the only chemical which glows in the dark. In contrast, UV tattoos are made up of dyes which fluoresce and are visible only under a black light. They do not glow in the dark. The color ranges from white to purple depending on the ink selected for the tattoo. The side effects are mainly due to the phosphorous inks which range from severe blistering, skin rashes to development of cancer.

THREE-DIMENSIONAL FX TRANSFERS TATTOO

The regular tattoos are 2D (two-dimensional). They are flat images with only height and width and lack depth. The term 3D (three-dimensional) tattoos

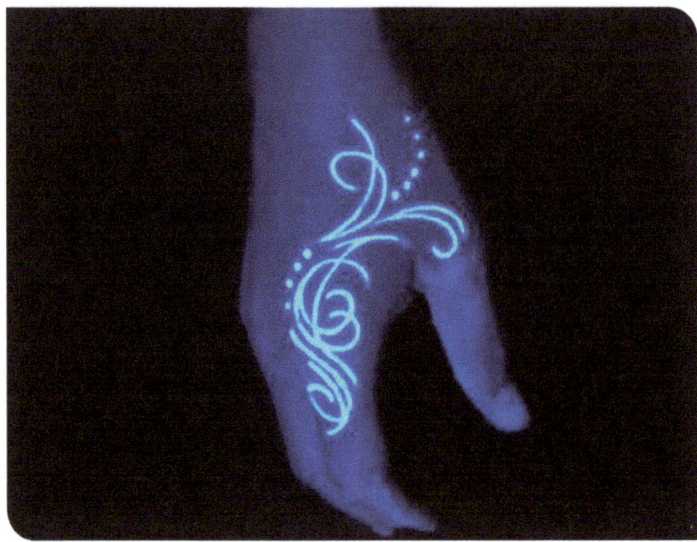

Fig. 9.11: Glow in the dark tattoos.

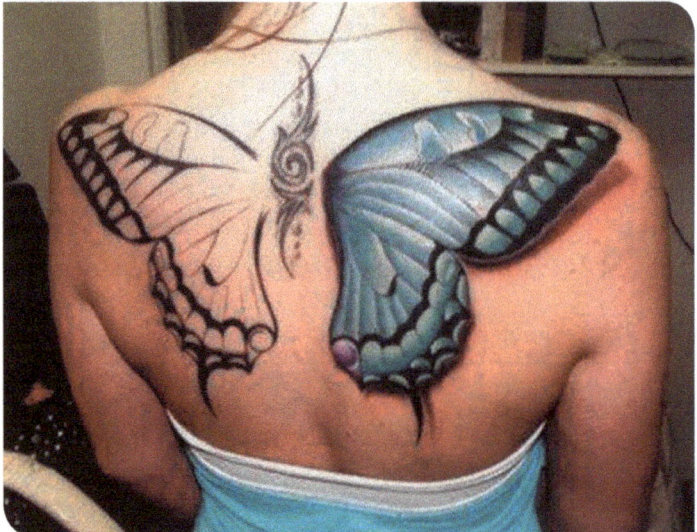

Fig. 9.12: Highlights the difference in 2D and 3D tattoos.

are used to indicate art and animation that uses an extra third dimension, i.e. the depth. It is this third dimension along with the shadows and shadings used by the tattoo artists which imparts a life-like effect to 3D tattoos. These tattoos are mainly used to create optical illusions.

Figure 9.12 highlights the difference in 2D and 3D tattoos. Left wing has no lighting and shadows; hence, it appears as an image on the skin. Right

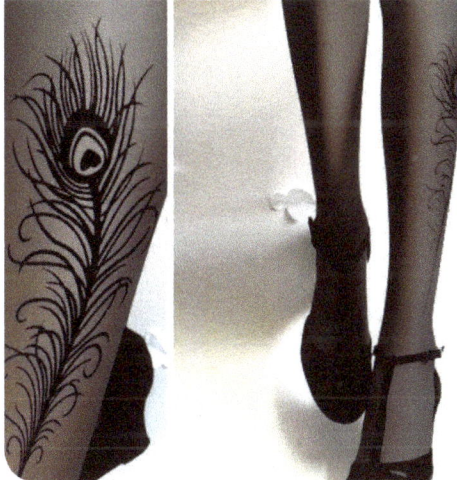

Fig. 9.13: Tattoo socks.

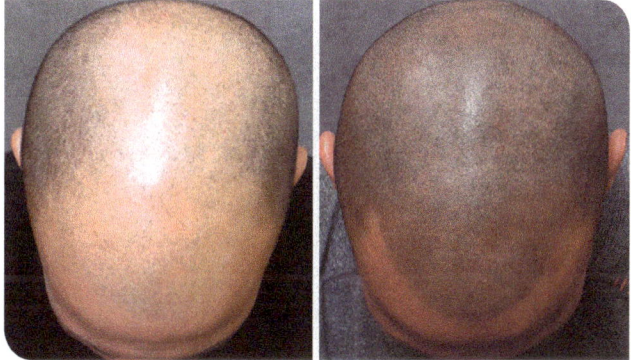

Fig. 9.14: Bald areas covered with tattoo inks.

wing has surface and shadows giving an illusion as though the butterfly wing is "above" the skin.

TATTOO SOCKS

This is another option for permanent and temporary tattoos. The socks which are worn as tights come in different designs like peacock feather, etc. (Fig. 9.13) that gives an illusion of a tattoo.

HAIR TATTOO

Also known as "scalp micropigmentation" is becoming popular nowadays as a cover-up remedy for baldness as shown in Figure 9.14. It gives a buzz cut hairstyle on a bald scalp. It is also used to cover up scars after hair transplantation and also create an illusion of thicker hairs if thinning of hairs is present. In contrast to regular tattoos the ink is not deeply incorporated into the scalp and is less prone for fading over years.

REFERENCES

1. Kazandjieva J, Grozdev I, Tsankov N. Temporary henna tattoos. Clin Dermatol. 2007;25:383-7.
2. Jung P, Sesztak-Greinecker G, Wantke F, et al. The extent of black henna tattoo's complications are not restricted to PPD-sensitization. Contact Dermatitis. 2006;55:57.
3. Perez RG, Gonzalez R, Gonzalez M, et al. Palpebral eczema due to contact allergy to henna used as a hair dye. Contact Dermatitis. 2003;48:238.
4. Lestringant GG, Bener A, Frossard PM. Cutaneous reactions to henna and associated additives. Br J Dermatol. 1999;141:598-600.
5. Dutta A, Malhotra S. Henna tattoo: an unusual peripheral venous access difficulty. J Anesth. 2010;24:321-2.
6. Kandil HH, Al-Ghanem MM, Sarwat MA, et al. Henna (Lawsonia inermis Linn.) inducing haemolysis among G6PD-deficient newborns. A new clinical observation. Ann Trop Paediatr. 1996;16:287-91.
7. Scibilia J, Galdi E, Biscaldi G, et al. Occupational asthma caused by black henna. Allergy. 1997;52:231-2.
8. de Groot AC. Side-effects of henna and semi-permanent 'black henna' tattoos: a full review. Contact Dermatitis. 2013;69(1):1-25.

Chapter 10

Tattoo Regulations

Umashankar Nagaraju

INTRODUCTION

Tattooing has become increasingly popular and fashionable all over the world particularly in the last decade. It is becoming increasingly fashionable even in India these days to have a tattoo, particularly among youngsters without having any basic education on contents of tattoo material and the requirement for sterility before getting the tattoo done.

This can result in the raising occurrence of complications and adverse reactions, some of them related to the procedures, other side effects caused by the substances used. In order to identify the causative agent it is essential to know the exact composition and nature of the materials applied. Improper and unhygienic practice may result in localized skin infections at the site of the tattoo or piercing. There is also the risk of transmission of blood-borne viruses, for example hepatitis B, hepatitis C, hepatitis D or human immunodeficiency virus (HIV), which can have more serious and long-term health consequences. It is therefore important that practitioners have safe working practices and particularly that good infection control practices are followed at all times, so that both clients and practitioners are protected.

There are no nationally recognized or accredited training courses, standards for practice, agreed knowledge and skills frameworks or arrangements for monitoring and reporting of professional competence. Although a lot of research has been done in this field, there is still a lack of uniform worldwide regulation on the procedures and materials. Tattoo compounds in comparison to cosmetics are in general not officially controlled. Moreover, the origin as well as the chemical and toxicological specifications of these coloring agents are hardly known by the producers, the performers, or even by the professionals involved in these procedures, and certainly not by the consumers.

INTERNATIONAL REGULATIONS

Tattoo inks and the pigments in these inks are considered as cosmetics and color additives and should be safe. Although some colorants are approved for use in cosmetics none is approved for injection into the skin. The Food and Drug Administration (FDA) does not strictly regulate and control these materials or the practice of tattooing, and in the United States of America (USA) these matters have been covered by local laws and jurisdictions mainly intended to regulate the body art establishments.[1] Although tattoo inks are implanted intradermally it would be reasonable to treat these products like medicine, concerning their sterility and composition. The Council of Europe (CoE) has dealt with the safety issue of tattooing for years and adopted in 2003 the CoE Resolution on the regulation of tattooing products.[2] Recently, Resolution ResAP(2008)[1] on requirements and criteria for the safety of tattoos [superseding Resolution ResAP(2003)[2] on tattoos and permanent makeup (PMU)] was adopted by the CoE and recommends that the governments of the member states take into account the principles set out in the resolution.[3] This resolution not only "follows a negative list approach by listing the substances which must not be used in tattooing products, based on current knowledge in this field", but also recommends "to regulate the use of substances in tattoos by taking steps toward establishing, on the basis of safety assessments carried out by competent bodies and harmonized at European level, an exhaustive list of substances proved safe for this use under certain conditions (positive list)". This resolution has already been implemented in the Dutch law. The resolution includes specifications about the content of the tattoo products, the labeling, the conditions of application and the obligation to inform the public and the consumer about the health risks of tattoos and tattooing practice.

For every ready-to-use product that is on the market under the European Union (EU) Cosmetics Directive, there should be a dossier to be held at the address mentioned in the product label. Any country can ask the "dossier-owning country" to consult the content of this dossier. All the products must be labeled and provided with an ingredient list that can be consulted by the consumer. Products that do not comply with the regulations cannot be sold lawfully and must be removed from the market. Competent surveillance authorities should be empowered by law to remove the product judged to pose a threat to the health of the consumer. Professionals should be obliged by law to check that only ready-to-use products complying with the regulation are used on their clients. The ultimate responsibilities are applicable to the producers, the authorities and professionals.[4]

From the medical perspective, this approach certainly offers opportunities to reduce the risks and complications involved in the use of chemical components that might be potentially hazardous and may threaten the health of the tattooed individual with special concern for heavy metals and carcinogenic aromatic amines; recommendations on the conditions of the application of tattoos should also minimize the risk of transmission of infectious diseases.[5]

The regulation of tattoo colors in the EU and Denmark is covered by general legislation regarding product safety. However, In India so far there is no such regulations. Tattooing and tattoo ink in India continue to be without any control of any significance by the authorities. At present, there are no rules about hygiene or preventive measures to limit the risks that are known at the time of tattoo for limiting the transfer of infections, including hepatitis and (rarely) syphilis. We need regulations to be followed with Indian perspective. The guidelines should emphasize the specifications for a toxicological safety assessment.

REASONS FOR FAILURE TO ENFORCE LAW IN EUROPE[2]

- There is a lack of research-based knowledge about tattoos. The deficit of knowledge especially affects the questions about the extent to which tattoo ink triggers allergy and phototoxicity, and whether the chemical substances in ink are carcinogenic, mutagenic and/or reproduction toxic to an extent that is clinically relevant. There is a lack of clinical and epidemiological knowledge as a rationale for regulation.
- None of the methods mentioned have been validated for analysis of tattoo pigments and ingredients. The resolution has proven to be difficult to implement because of the lack of precision of the analysis techniques and test methods, but also because of the extensive requirements that the manufacturers are not currently able to comply with. Another weakness is that it has not been possible to relate the critical constituent substances to the tattoo complications that are observed in the clinic. There is a lack of knowledge about the release of tattoo ink's chemical substances in the skin and systemically in people who are tattooed. The knowledge about the substances' biokinetics from animal experiments has only been studied in some mouse studies, which cannot provide the basis for conclusions about exposure in human situations. Finally, the resolution is of limited significance because the tattoo ink that is in the market is manufactured based on large number of pigments, chemical variations and decomposition substances. Chemical quality assurance of tattoo ink is, therefore, very complex and difficult due to the large number of constituent substances and their possibilities for chemical and toxicological effect and interference.
- The CoA's resolution has not succeeded in solving the problem of the microbial safety of tattoo ink. In this area, there is a great deal of basic knowledge and clarity about unwanted microbial agents, the reasons for

complications and their manifestation in the form of systemic infection and danger to the tattooed person.

THE NATIONAL TATTOO ASSOCIATION: NEED OF THE HOUR

The law to be implemented similar to one in Denmark (The Act of 1966 was supplemented by a new act on tattooing that was adopted by the Danish Parliament on May 1, 2013[6]) so that the tattooists are registered voluntarily through the National Tattooists Associations, as a kind of quality control of the ink use, and a requirement that ink must be sterile. Such association should be formally approved by the Government of India, Department of Health and Family Welfare. The association takes care of education and the determination of rules as a prerequisite for the tattooists being registered.

KEY FACTORS TO BE CONSIDERED FOR GUIDELINES

- There are 20 aromatic amines on the negative list due to their potential carcinogenic, mutagenic, reproductive toxic and sensitizing properties. The tattoo artists must be aware of these.
- The main emphasis of the guidelines should be on the preparation of the safety assessment and the safety report. The safety report must establish that the tattoo color does not present a risk to human health when tattooing. This is ensured by using information about the tattoo products' safety and also a safety assessment of the information. Thus, there must be a thorough toxicological account regarding all of the constituent substances in the product, including impurities. Exposure risks regarding the product, as well as substances and mixes, including impurities, must also be stated.

GUIDELINES PROPOSED BY THE AUTHOR FOR CONSIDERATION BY THE REGULARIZING AUTHORITY OF INDIA

- *Age limits:* Only people who are 18 years of age or older should be tattooed.
- Tattoo colors should be covered by the law on chemical substances and products and the product safety law. The resolution should ensure to mention about the expiry dates of tattoo ink.
- *Consent form:* The signing of a declaration and providing proof of age should be a fundamental part of the client consultation process and

practitioners should always require that the client signs a consent form prior to any work being commenced. However, the consent will only be valid, if the customer has been fully informed as to the nature of the process, the likely effect and potential problems involved. For practitioners own protection, it is recommended that any consent forms they use are worded with the advice of a solicitor who is familiar with this area of law.

- *Registration requirements for tattoo parlors/shops*:
  - No person, firm, partnership or corporation should describe its services in any manner under the title "tattoo" unless such services as defined herein are performed in a parlor/shop that is registered with the Department of Health and Family Welfare. The Department of Health shall be responsible for the administrative functions required to implement the rules and regulations herein, as they apply to the registering of tattoo parlors/shops.
  - No person shall engage in the practice of tattooing or hold himself/herself as a tattoo artist unless he/she is registered under the statutory and regulatory provisions herein. Provided, that physicians duly licensed to practice medicine shall be exempt from this registration requirement.
  - Any applicant seeking registration must: (a) be over 18 years of age, and (b) be of good moral character.
  - Applicants seeking registration as a tattoo artist shall be required to demonstrate aseptic tattooing technique via an examination administered by the Department of Health and Family Welfare.
  - *Renewal:* Said registration, unless sooner suspended or revoked, shall expire by limitation on particular day of the year following its issuance and may be renewed from year to year after inspection and/or approval by the registration agency, provided the applicant meets the appropriate statutory and regulatory requirements herein.
  - A registration shall be issued only to a specific applicant for a specific location, and shall not be transferable.
  - *Inspections:* Duly authorized representatives of the registration agency shall, at all reasonable times, have the authority to enter upon any and all parts of the premises on which any tattoo parlor/shop is located to make any investigation or inspection to determine conformity with the statutory and regulatory provisions herein.
  - The registering authority is authorized to deny an application, or revoke a registration for cause (e.g. conviction of crimes) or for failure of an applicant or registrant to comply with the provisions of these rules and regulations. The applicant or registrant shall be given an opportunity for a prompt and fair hearing in accordance with the provisions of law.

- Dyes, pigments, and stencils:
  - All dyes and pigments shall be manufactured for the purpose of tattooing and used according to the manufacturer's specifications.
  - In preparing dyes or pigments, nontoxic materials shall be used.
  - Single-use, sterile, individual containers for dyes or pigments shall be used for each client.
  - The stencil, unless composed of acetate, shall be used for a single tattoo procedure only.
  - Acetate stencils may be disinfected and reused.
- *Tattoo procedures:* A tattoo artist shall conduct his/her tattooing practice so as to prevent the transmission of communicable diseases from client to client and from artist to client. Tattoo artists shall maintain atleast the following minimum standards in the practice of tattooing:
  - The area of the body to be tattooed, and all parts of the body which are visible, shall be examined for signs of intravenous drug use, open sores, lesions, oozing wounds, and skin diseases. If such are found, or suspected, the person shall not be tattooed.
  - Each tattoo artist shall wear a clean outer garment. If the garment is visibly contaminated with blood, it shall be changed between clients.
  - Before working on each client, each tattoo artist shall clean his/her own fingernails with a brush and shall thoroughly wash and scrub hands with hot running water, using germicidal soap from a dispenser. Hands must also be washed after each rest room use, before putting on gloves and after taking off gloves.
- Tattoo materials:
  - All materials necessary for the tattooing process shall be set up on a single-use disposable sterile cloth (e.g. polycloth). All autoclaved/ sterile packs shall be opened ready for use without touching the interior of the pack.
  - Any shaving shall be done with a single-use razor blade or razor.
  - The skin shall be prepared first by thoroughly soaping with an antiseptic soap and rinsing with tap water. Following this cleansing, a germicidal solution (such as 70% isopropyl alcohol) shall be applied to the skin using a sterile swab.
  - After applying the stencil, the tattoo artist shall remove and discard gloves and again wash and scrub his/her hands with soap and water and dry hands using paper towels.
  - Prior to commencing application of the tattoo, the tattoo artist shall then put on sterile gloves, which shall be used for a single tattooing procedure only.
  - If there is a need to rinse the tube and needle between colors, this shall be done with 91% isopropyl alcohol or sterile water in sterile single-use disposable containers or nondisposable sterilized containers.

- The tattoo shall be allowed to dry. After drying, a sterile lubricant shall be applied from a collapsible metal or plastic tube, and the entire area covered with a piece of sterile gauze.
- Needles shall be immediately deposited into a puncture-resistant infectious waste sharps container. Needles shall not be reused.
- All used needles and any blood soaked material shall be handled and discarded according to the *Rules and Regulations of Biomedical Waste Management*. All other material shall be discarded appropriately.
- All tubes and line bars must be rinsed with tap water and then placed in a germicidal solution (e.g. Cidex) or directly into an ultrasonic cleaner.
- Sterile gloves shall be removed and discarded in accordance with the requirements of the *Rules and Regulations of Biomedical Waste Management*.
- Immediately after tattooing, the tattoo artist shall advise the client both verbally and in writing-on the care of the tattoo and shall instruct the client to consult a dermatologist at the first sign of infection (such as excessive pain, redness, swelling, or discharge) in the area of the tattoo.
- All work surfaces and nonautoclaved equipment (e.g. tattoo machine and pliers) used in the tattoo process shall be cleaned with bactericidal, virucidal, fungicidal, tuberculocidal surface disinfectant/decontaminant cleaner between clients. Gloves shall be used in the cleaning process. Subsequently, the artist shall wash his/her hands with a germicidal soap after cleaning work surfaces and equipment.
- After tattooing, the remaining unused dye or pigment shall be discarded in accordance with the requirements of the *Rules and Regulations of Biomedical Waste Management*.
- *Tattoo equipment*:
  - A set of individual, single-use sterilized needle bars shall be used for each new client. Before each use, the open end of the needle tube of the tattooing machine shall be cleaned and sterilized in an approved manner.
  - Adequate numbers of sterilized needles and tubes shall be on hand for each operator for the entire day or night operation, based on the average number of clients per day. Failure to maintain an adequate number of sterilized needles and tubes shall require the artist to cease operations until such time as an adequate number becomes available.
  - Storage cabinets shall be maintained in a sanitary condition and all instruments, dyes, pigments, stencils and other equipment, when not in use, shall be stored in an orderly manner.
- *Sterilizing of instruments*:
  - Operational sterilizers shall be available in each tattoo parlor and used appropriately.

- Autoclave units shall be checked monthly, using a standard spore test, with results maintained on file for inspection. Autoclave units shall be maintained in accordance with manufacturer's specifications. Records of said monthly checks shall be maintained for a minimum of 2 years.
- A log book shall be maintained for the results of said monthly inspections and shall include no less than the following items: date of inspection, results of inspection, and the signature of the tattoo artist who conducted the inspection.
- The sterilizing date shall be noted, and evidence of sterilization shall be demonstrated by color indicator or equivalent. Packs shall be used within 30 days or resterilized.
- *Personnel*:
  - Each facility shall submit to the registration agency:
    - The name of the owner and/or manager who shall be responsible for the management and control of the operation and the maintenance of the facility.
    - The facility's conformity with state and local laws and regulations pertaining to fire, safety, building sanitation, personnel and other relevant statutory and regulatory provisions, and
    - The establishment of policies and procedures, including but not limited to, the practice of tattooing, sanitation protocols, infection control, the nature of services provided and other such policies and procedures as may be required.
  - Persons engaged in the practice of tattooing shall comply with the Occupational Safety and Health Administration's (OSHA) Bloodborne Pathogens Standard in order to protect themselves (and any employees) against occupational exposure to bloodborne pathogens.[7]
  - Compliance shall include, but not be limited to:
    - A written exposure control plan
    - Staff training
    - Engineering and work practice controls
    - Adoption of universal precautions
    - Personal protective equipment
    - Hepatitis B vaccinations, and
    - A protocol for evaluation in the event that an exposure occurs.
- *Environment and maintenance:* Each tattoo parlor/shop shall be required to meet the following provisions:
  - The facility shall be maintained in a sanitary condition free from hazards.
  - All walls, ceilings, and floors shall be smooth and easily cleanable and have a nonabsorbent surface. There shall be no carpeting in the tattooing area. Walls and ceilings are to be painted in a light color. Walls, ceilings and floors shall be kept clean and in good repair, free from

dust and debris. Floors, walls or ceilings shall not be swept or cleaned while tattooing is being performed.

- Adequate light and ventilation shall be provided.
- Each tattoo parlor/shop shall contain a hand sink in the tattooing area for the exclusive use of the tattoo artist. The sink shall have hot and cold running water. At the sink, there shall also be available: a soap dispenser, disposable towels and refuse containers.
- In facilities in which there are multiple tattooing workstations, there shall be a minimum of one sink per every two workstations.
- All work surfaces shall be smooth, nonporous and easily cleanable.
- The facility shall be arranged so that work areas are separated from waiting customers by providing a separate room for tattooing or by providing at least ten feet between work areas and partitioning the areas with panels (or other barriers) at least six feet high. The panel may be constructed of solid opaque plastic or similar material.
- Equipment and supplies shall be properly stored in designated storage cabinets.
- No smoking, eating or drinking shall be permitted in the tattooing area.
- *Waste disposal:* Medical waste shall be managed in accordance with the *Rules and Regulations of Biomedical Waste Management.*
- *Retention of records:* The owner of a tattooing parlor/shop shall maintain proper records for each client. A record of each client shall include:
  - The date on which he/she was tattooed
  - His/her name, address, telephone number and age; photo identification as proof of age, a copy of which shall be maintained for each client
  - The location and design of the tattoo, and
  - The name of the tattoo artist.

These records shall be permanently entered in a book with prenumbered pages, kept solely for this purpose. These records shall be available for inspection by the Department of Health. These records shall be maintained for a minimum of 5 years after the date on which the client was tattooed.

TATTOO POLICY FOR CANDIDATES APPEARING FOR SERVICES SELECTION BOARD (SSB) INTERVIEW FOR ARMY WITH PERMANENT BODY TATTOO(S)[8]

The Tattoo Policy has been revised recently and the new policy was implemented with effect from May 11, 2015. Some of the salient aspects:
- Tattoo site:
  - *Candidates from tribal communities:* Candidates belonging to tribal communities/from tribal areas, as declared by the Government

of India Scheduled Castes and Scheduled Tribes Orders Act/Lists (amended and modified from time to time), are permitted to have permanent body tattoos on any part of the body, as per existing customs and traditions of the said tribe to which a candidate belongs.

- *All other candidates:* Permanent body tattoos are permitted on the following body parts only, for which a candidate will be required to sign a Self-Certification Certificate:
    - Inner part (medial) of forearms, i.e. from inside of the elbow to the wrist of both the hands (area between 1–2 and 3 in picture affixed). Note: Area between 4, 5, and 6 is not permitted (Fig. 10.1A).
    - Reverse side of the palm/back (dorsal) side of both hands (area between 2 and 3 in picture affixed) (Fig. 10.1B).
- Nature of tattoos:
    - *Permissible tattoos*:
        - Though no restriction on size or type of tattoo has been specified, tattoos are only permitted on body parts as mentioned earlier.
        - Only small innocuous tattoos, that are not prejudicial to good order and military discipline are permitted, e.g. religious symbols or names of near and dear ones, etc.
    - *Nonpermissible tattoos:* Regardless of location of a tattoo on the body (permitted/not permitted), the following will fall under the category of "nonpermissible tattoos":
        - Tattoos on any other part of the body (less mentioned earlier).
        - A tattoo with lewd or offensive content or indecent figures.
        - Tattoos that are indecent, sexist or racist, explained as follows:
            ◦ Indecent tattoos are those that are grossly offensive to modesty, decency or propriety.
            ◦ Sexist tattoos are those that advocate a philosophy that demeans a person based on gender.
            ◦ Racist tattoos advocate a philosophy that degrades or demeans a person based on race, ethnicity or region and religion.

ACCEPTANCE/NONACCEPTANCE OF PERMANENT BODY TATTOO(S)

Any candidate with a permanent body tattoo(s) on any part of the body other than that specified earlier (permissible category), or is of an objectionable nature (nonpermissible category), as brought out earlier, *are not eligible for enrolment into the Armed Forces.*

In case a candidate has undergone removal of tattoo(s) prior to appearing for Services Selection Board (SSB) interview and the same has faded substantially, this will be treated as a "scar" and not a tattoo. Such candidates

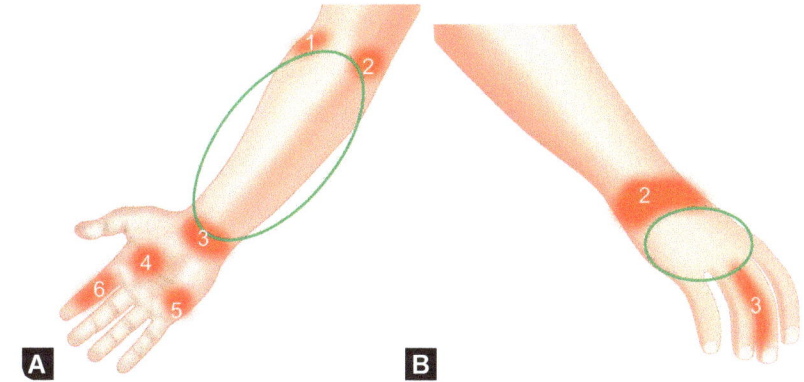

Figs. 10.1A and B: (A) Parts where permanent body tattoos can be tattooed (area between 1–2 and 3). Note: Area between 4, 5, and 6 is not permitted for permanent body tattoos. (B) Permanent body tattoos can be tattooed between area 2 and 3.

will be permitted to undergo the entire selection process subject to approval by the Commandant, Selection Center.

TATTOO AND BLOOD DONATION

There is no strict law or policy on blood donation in person with tattoo in India. But Indian red cross society recommends individuals to wait for six months to be eligible for blood donation if piercing or tattoo were performed under safe sanitary conditions (sterile or disposable equipment). Otherwise, they are deferred for one year. But the screening investigations are continued as with other donors.

TATTOO AND ORGAN DONATIONS

Again no enforcing law in India but organ donations is deferred for 1 year after tattooing.

CONCLUSION

The increasing popularity of body adornment through piercing and tattooing in its different forms has raised many questions about the safety of the techniques and the materials used. Many efforts have been done yet to identify the risk factors and to develop preventive measures aimed at protecting public health. Regulation of the composition of the products, harmonization of the methods for the analytical determination of possible harmful substances and recommendations to ensure that procedures are carried out under appropriate hygienic conditions offer a big step forward to promoting consumers health.

REFERENCES

1. De Cuyper C, D'hollander D. Materials used in body art. In: De Cuyper C, Pérez-Cotapos SM (Eds). Dermatologic Complications with Body Art. Germany: Springer-Verlag; 2010. pp. 13-28.
2. The Council of Europe. (2003). Resolution ResAP(2003)2 on tattoos and permanent make-up. [online] Available from rm.coe.int/CoERMPublicCommon SearchServices/DisplayDCTMContent?documentId=09000016805df8e5. [Accessed April, 2017].
3. Council of Europe. (2008). ResAP(2008)1. [online] Available from https://wcd.coe.int/ViewDoc. [Accessed April, 2017].
4. Talberg HJ. The question of positive or negative lists. In: Papameletiou D, Schwela D, Zenie A, Baeumler W (Eds). Workshop on the Technical/Scientific and Regulatory Issues on the Safety of Tattoos, Body Piercing and Related Practices. Ispra: European Commission; 2003. pp. 84-8.
5. Serup J, Harrit N, Linnet JT, et al. Tattoos - Health, Risks and Culture. With an Introduction to the "Seamless Prevention" Strategy. Copenhagen: The Council on Health and Disease Prevention; 2015. pp. 1-156.
6. Retsinformation.dk. (2013). Lov om en frivillig, brancheadministreret regis-treringsordning for tatovører [Danish action voluntary industry-administered registration programme for tattooists]. [online] Available from www.retsinfor-mation.dk/Forms/R0710.aspx-?id=146551. [Accessed April, 2017].
7. Occupational Safety and Health Administration (OSHA). (1992). Intro to 29 CFR Part 1910, Occupational Exposure to Bloodborne Pathogens. [online] Available from www.osha.gov/pls/oshaweb/owadisp.show_document?p_table= PREAMBLES&p_id=801. [Accessed April, 2017].
8. Indian Army. (2015). Tattoo policy for candidates appearing for SSB interview with permanent body tattoo(s). [online] Available from joinindianarmy.nic.in/writereaddata/Portal/Images/pdf/tattopolicy2015.pdf. [Accessed April, 2017].

Index

Note: Page numbers followed by *f* refer to figure and *t* refer to table.

www.ingramcontent.com/pod-product-compliance
Lightning Source LLC
Chambersburg PA
CBHW041345210526
45162CB00014B/4